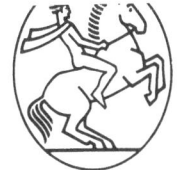

Language and Speech

Proceedings of the Fifth Convention
of the Academia Eurasian Neurochirurgica
Budapest, September 19–22, 1990

Edited by
E. Pásztor, J. Vajda, and F. Loew

Acta Neurochirurgica
Supplementum 56

Springer-Verlag Wien New York

Professor Emil Pásztor, M.D.
János Vajda, M.D.
National Institute of Neurosurgery, Budapest, Hungary

Professor Friedrich Loew, M.D.
Neurochirurgische Universitätsklinik, Homburg/Saar, Federal Republic of Germany

With 46 Figures

Typesetting: Thomson Press, New Delhi, India

Printed on acid-free paper

ISSN 0065-1419
ISBN 978-3-7091-9241-2   ISBN 978-3-7091-9239-9 (eBook)
DOI 10.1007/978-3-7091-9239-9

Preface

This time again, one of the great European cities hosts the coming convention of the Academy which bridges our continents. For the first time we will gather in Eastern Europe, in a country of changing socialism, and other systems represented.

According to the principles of the Academy, for this Convention we have selected a theme which is of great importance in neurosurgery, in neurophysiology, and is, at the same time, a fundamental entity in arts, history, philosophy; this theme is, language and speech.

It is the language, the most human aspect of interpersonal communication, which connects and divides our nations. Your host country, has a language which is, in fact, an island in the sea of languages. That has produced hardship in all periods for Hungary and has isolated her from other nations.

It is now hoped that lectures, discussions and informal exchange of ideas in a colourful environment of warm hospitality will further tighten our unity and enrich everyone who joins us.

E. Pásztor   J. Vajda

Contents

Hutterer, C.J.: Prelogical Relics in Language Development 1

Ujfalussy, J.: The Role of Music and Song in Human Communication 6

Ádám, G.: Communication in Animals 9

Nádasdy, Á.: Language Families 14

Szentágothai, J.: Functional Anatomy of Human Speech 17

Altenmüller, E., Kriechbaum, W., Helber, U., Moini, S., Dichgans, J., Petersen, D.: Cortical
    DC-Potentials in Identification of the Language-Dominant
    Hemisphere: Linguistical and Clinical Aspects 20

Friberg, L.: Brain Mapping in Thinking and Language Function 34

Lebrun, Y., Leleux, C.: The Effects of Electrostimulation and of Resective and Stereotactic Surgery on
    Language and Speech 40

Kertesz, A.: Clinical Forms of Aphasia 52

Ramamurthi, B., Chari, P.: Aphasia in Bilinguals 59

Tandon, P., Mahapatra, A.K., Khosla, A.: Operations on Gliomas Involving Speech Centres 67

Adams, C.B.T.: The Surgery for Epilepsy with Speech Arrest 72

Srinivasan, K.: Lateralisation of Speech Centre in Left-Handedness Due to Cerebral
    and Extracerebral Lesions 83

Osman-Sági, J.: Psychological Mechanisms of Speech Rehabilitation in Aphasic Patients 85

Lovász, L.: Features of Computer Language: Communication of Computers and Its Complexity 91

Vámos, T.: Computer and the Thought Process 96

Listed in Current Contents

Acta Neurochirurgica (1993) [Suppl] 56: 1–5

Prelogical Relics in Language Development

C.J. Hutterer

Department of German Language and Literature Karl-Franzens-Universität, Graz, Austria

1. The technical term *prelogic, prelogical* (thinking) was established by the French philosopher and ethnograph Lucien Lévy-Bruhl (1857–1939) and it means that by primitive man "collective ideas" were not thought according to the rules of formal logic, on the contrary, the rise of such ideas about the surroundings of man was throughout "prelogical", i.e. distinct from logical thinking in modern sense and in no way directed by the rules of formal logic.

Philosophy was at its beginnings in ancient Greece, a philosophy of language closely depending on the growth of man's knowledge about reality. Fundamental terms of logic like *subject, object, predicate* etc., which became defined by Aristotle and other Greek philosophers on the background of language, were all along the line first-rate tools of man in understanding and – what is more – in the interpretation of the world. But the development of knowledge has ever been a long-winded and tiresome, step-by-step process, and new perceptions were bound by systemized grammatical and semantical frameworks of human languages. So the further development of human logic has ever been handicapped by a sort of dilatoriness. That is why the realization of a *rational grammar* turns out to be impossible and why philosophers of the Vienna school, in particular Wittgenstein, became astonished – as they thought – by such a moment of inertia in language.

One of the founders of modern linguistics, a close friend and fellow of Wilhelm v. Humboldt, Hans Connon von der Gabelentz said in his work about passive forms in several languages more than hundred years ago that language does not express what is to be presented, only the personal ideas of the speaker(s); in this sense language cannot be objective and it gives back an image of reality in the speakers' mind. We can point out that language is no mathematical system and therefore it has no "logic" once and for all. Logic in language is developing according to the mental evolution of the native speakers of every natural language. As a system once having been constituted by convention it cannot be changed at once and so it must follow the mental evolution of its speakers with a relevant difference in time and in its form.

By way of illustration just an example: Today we know that the Earth is not the centre of our solar system and the sun does not revolve round our globe, but on the contrary, our globe rotates round the sun as the centre of our solar system. Notwithstanding we are accustomed to say "the sun rises", "the sun sets" – and it is so in other languages too. It is similar, but anyway more difficult in a problem like words as *soothsayer* = Germ. *Wahrsager*. In this case we must believe in occultism and have an almost religious faith that people exist who know what is to be or come to pass as a reality.

By the way, etymology shows that we are always speaking in metaphors and we are always linking one thing to another. An innocent word as *(to) see* = Germ. *sehen* originally means "to follow" and is related to Latin *sequor*. In Germanic it meant "to follow with the eyes", i.e. "to see" in our present usage. *To sleep* = Germ. *schlafen* is related to Latin *labio* "to glide". In Germanic it came to be used in the sense "to glide over from a state of wakefulness to that of unconsciousness". Such expressions and words are well functioning but logically they are incorrect, even prelogical.

Here it is not possible to trace the question in its relations down to the smallest detail. I am going to review a modest collection of specimens in several languages which are still dragging the heritage of ancient times when their speakers had quite another view upon things and beings than we have today.

2. One of the first steps in language development was the try-out of primitive man to determine qualification and – much later – quantification of his environment. By and by he learned to differentiate between objects and actions and moreover between diverse types of objects and actions. Certainly, this step was headed towards logical systematization of creatures and things, but just at the given level of man"s knowledge.

For a possible ancestral way of classification in modern languages we can refer to one of the most important vernaculars of Africa, to Swahili. Semantical classification of words as well as their changes come in Swahili at the beginning of the words. The most relevant class is the so called *M-WA*-class (or *WATU*-class, meaning "people") denoting persons. The nouns of this class make their plural with the prefix *WA*, e.g. *mtu* "man" > *watu* "men, people", *mtoto* "child" > *watoto* "children" and this prefix characterizes syntagmatic groups as a whole: *watu warefu wawili* "two tall men" (*refu* "long", *wili* "two"). The *WATU*-class involves animals too: *ndege* "bird" + *zuri* "good" > *ndege wazuri* "pretty birds". Things belong to the *KI*-class (plural prefix: *VI-*) and this class forms from the root *-tu* (as above) the word *KItu* "thing", in plural *VItu* "things". This elementary difference to "beings" and "things" we meet in very differnt languages. But Swahili moved on and shaped up analogical classification prefixes for properties and abstractions, e.g. *U-tu* "manhood", *JI-tu* "a huge man" (> *MAJItu* "huge men") etc.

This mechanism may be curious for speakers thinking in IE. (= Indo-European) categories. However, an older stage of development reveals also in English, German, Latin or Slavic etc. a method very similar to that of Swahili. Many languages of Indo-European made/make a difference between animate and inanimate phenomena, e.g. in Russian inflexion of nouns no formal difference appears between nominative and accusative if they are neutral: *čelovek* > *čeloveka* "man: Nom. > Acc.", but *dom* > *dom* "house: Nom. > Acc.". It is well-known that in Latin, neutral nouns – originally meaning inanimate things or animals – nominative and accusative have the same form: *pater* > *patrem* masc., *mater* > *matrem* fem., but *bellum* "war" (nom.-acc.), *animal* (nom.-acc.). The background of this distinction is simple: words being classified as neuters were thought as objects of any action only, but never as subjects, i.e. actors of an action. This stage already represented a further step on the way of classification.

Quite anciently we can bring a type to light coinciding with Swahili prefixation. A good example of it is found in the so called *s mobile* in IE. languages. As an old prefix this *s* was or even is connected with many roots meaning (primitive) actors in some languages, while it is missing in some other related languages. So we find it in English *steer* "a young castrated ox; any male of beef cattle" like *Stier* "bull" in German, but not in Latin *taurus* ~ Greek *tauros* "bull" nor in Slavic *tur* "bison ibex". Otherwise the root being revealed in English *murder* and German *Mord* exist in Russian quasi personified in *s-mert'* "death" with an *s mobile*. It can be supposed that the same *s* appears in such "action" forms of the verb *to be* which are derivated, e.g. *is* (Germ. *ist*), Lat. *sunt* ~ Germ. *sind* etc., likewise in the nominal flexion in Latin nominative/genitive ending like *dominus, patris patres* etc., or in Saxon genitive in English (*man's*, Germ. *Mannes*).

We see that animate-inanimate differentiation was ahead of the differentiation according to genders of the nouns. But also this classification in conformity of genders is today an overhang in modern logical sense (cf. *das Weib, das Mädchen* in German, *child* as a neuter and *man-of-war* or *ship* as a feminine word in English!) In these languages such a classification has become a mixture of *sex* and grammatical *gender* and is oscillating on the border of semantics and grammar. In a logical sense this distinction is unnecessary.

Such mixed distinctions can be very complicated: in Asmat – a Papuan language in New Guinea – we find 5 classes: one for "standing" phenomena (as trees, people etc. which are thin and high), another for "sitting" phenomena (as houses, women etc. which are tall and broad), a third one for "lying" phenomena (as trees being cut down or little animals which are broad and small or short, but also the words for the rising sun as like as for the rising moon), the fourth class involves "swimming" phenomena (as fishes, boats and rivers), while the fifth class is reserved for "flying" phenomena (birds, insects and objects hanging or lying above).

3. A world-wide known ancient and primitive techniqe of languages is the repetition of words either to intensify the meaning or to give them another grammatical or semantical function. With the help of this reduplication we produce in English an increasing intensity saying e.g. *long-long ago* in the way as Malays in *lama-lama dahulu* (*lama* "long"). Full reduplication indicates plural forms of nouns in Malay too, e.g. *orang* "man" > *orang-orang* "men, people" (written very economically as *orang*[2]) or even a new meaning of the word: *mata* "eye" > *mata-mata* "1. eyes; 2. policeman"

(in the second case also partially reduplicated: *mĕmata*). Reduplication can be used to derive verbs from nouns in all Melanesian and Polynesian languages like Marshallese *wit* "flower" > *witwit* "to wear a flower". In the languages of the Pacific full reduplication seems to weaken the meaning, e.g. *wera* "hot" > *werawera* warm"; the partial reduplication has either the same effect (*pango* "black" > *papango* "dark") or indicates plurality (*roa* "long" in sing., *roroa* in plur. "the long ones"). In Dakota (= Sioux) reduplication strengthens the meaning: *sapa* "black" > *sapsapa* "quite black", *tehanyan* "far, long" > *tehanhanyan* "very far/long". Also in superlative expressing the extreme degree of comparison of adjectives and adverbs Dakota uses reduplication: *waxte* "good" > *waxtewaxte* "the best". In the languages of IE. origin reduplication is/was in use too, cf. Lat. *dedi* "I have given" from *do* "I give", and similarly in Greek verbal system. Germanic languages possess some relics only, but in Gothic reduplication was at the peak of its development in a separate group of verbs like *letan* "to let" > *lailot* in preterite.

4. All Germanic languages have a curious group of verbs, the so called preterito-present verbs. These verbs express present meanings in their historical preterite forms like Germ. *ich weiß* "I know" (Archaic Engl. *I wot*) or Engl. *may, can* etc. How is one to explain this "illogical" anomaly in the recent system of these languages? The mechanism I shall try to demonstrate by using the example of Archaic Engl. *I wot* ~ Germ. *ich weiß*. (By the way: the root itself is still existing in Engl. *to wit* and its derivates as *witless, witness, witted* etc.) Old Germanic *wait* "I know" goes back to IE. **woid-/*weid-/*wid-* in the meaning "to see, to catch sight of something" and this primary meaning we find in Lat. *video* "I see" or in Russ. *videt'* to "see" just as in the Greek aorist *eîdon* "I saw/perceived". The change of the meaning to that of knowing we find in Greek *oĩda* "to know" as well as in Sanskrit *véda*, too. The explanation for this change is simple enough and could be called as *ex post facto*; in a term of philosophy it is a *post-hoc*-relation: I know something or somebody after having seen it or him. From a stylistic point of view we are confronted with an evidence opposed to what has been said a *praesens historicum* with the difference that preterito-present verbs are no phenomena of style but are involved in the grammatical system of those languages. In any case they represent a former stage of "logicality".

In this connection let me mention another somehow strange feature of Germ.-IE. verbs. It is well known that from the preterite form of so called strong verbs (and form nouns) weak verbs can be derived expressing causation like *to fell* from *to fall* ("causatives"). In this way, from the Gothic preterito-present verb *lais* "I know" the weak verb *laisjan* could be derived meaning "to teach". It existed in Old Engl. as *lǣran* and still exists in Germ. *lehren* "to teach". Now, Gothic had a further "trick" in building new words. Parallel to those verbs with the suffix *-j-an* it also formed verbs with another suffix, the suffix *-n-an* to express passivity of the same action, e.g. in addition to *fulljan* "to fill" also *fullnan* "to be filled". In this way Gothic *laisnan* – like Engl. *learn* and Germ. *lernen* – originally do not mean an active process but a passive one: to *learn* means in Old Germanic thinking "to be put or caused to be in a position/situation of knowing", quite contrary to our modern thinking, as *learning* is in our understanding an active process.

5. The primary group of Germanic verbs – that of the "strong" verbs – form several tenses from several stem variants of the same root by apophony, i.e. with the help of vowel changes in the roots like *drink > drank > drunk* etc. Such verbs can be classified as several classes but all classes go back to the vowel change IE. *e ~ o* (as in Lat. *tego* "I cover/envelop" > *toga* "garment in ancient Rome, to-day a robe of office"). While in most IE. languages apophony serves as a relevant means in word formation; it also became in Germanic an important element in the build-up of grammatical forms, even verb roots. There are lots of proposals trying to explain the evolution of apophony and one of these seems to support our theory of prelogical relics in human speech. This proposal is concerned in the well-known phenomenon that with physically equal noises and sounds at a close range our hearing receives/ realizes as high, but as dull and low from afar. This way of perception becoming aware of acoustic impressions through the sense of hearing is a natural effect and by no means restricted to Germanic or IE. languages; it is a language universal indeed. Lat. *hic* "this" and *hīc* "here" versus *hoc* "that" and *hōc/hūc* "hither (from afar)" have their counterparts in Hungarian (a language of Fenno-Ugric origin) in words like *itt* "here" and *ott* "there", *ide* "hither" and *oda* "there: to that place". In Dakota (= Sioux), an Indian language of North America, two definite articles exist: *ki(n)* in connection with a person or thing that we see at the moment of use; *ko(n)* if we do not see it (therefore with preterite forms of verbs, too). In Wolof (a Senegalese-Guinean language in Africa) the article serving like Engl. *the*, but affixed to the noun has four forms regarding the distance from the speaker: *bāye* "father",

bāye-bi "the father (here)", *bāye-bu* "the father (there, but relatively near to the speaker), *bāye-bä* "the father" (relatively distant from the speaker) and *bāye-bā* "the father" (absolutely distant). Maybe, a similar way of perception lies in the vowel changes in Japanese *fito* "one" versus *futa* "two", *mi* "three" versus *mu* "six" as well as in *yo* "four" versus *ya* "eight".

For the natural effect of apophony we can also refer to onomatopoeia in Germanic languages. Engl. *ding-dong* as well as Germ. *bim-bam*, both for the sound of a bell struck repeatedly or for any similar sound stand all demands of apophonic rules in these languages and have their lexical derivates, e.g. in Engl. *to ding* as well as in *ding, dong* and in Germ. *bimmeln* "to tinkle", *bammeln/baumeln* "to dangle, swing", *bummeln* "to stroll, dawdle, loaf" and in interjections as *bum(m)!*, *bums!*, "boom!, bang!"

For our purpose it is especially significant that in Germanic strong verbs the form being acoustically perceived as "far-sounded" for the speakers is the *past* tense form (*sung* from *sing*, *drank*, *drunk* from *drink* and so on). We may find out that from an Old Germanic point of view present tense at first was realized as the next one, and only in the relation to it, i.e. secondly, a past tense as a "far one" in time (and space) could be developed. The ability to think in the future came up after thinking in present and past categories and accordingly the forming of a new tense for future events was the last one in Germanic – and, maybe, in every other – grammar of man. Old Germanic – like other language groups and families – had only two tenses: present and past and for long the present form also served at the same time as a future tense. All periphrastic forms of the future tense (*I shall/will come, ich werde kommen* etc.) are relatively modern acquisitions of these languages instead of the present form also in the grammatical sense of futurity.

6. Today we are thrown upon numbers or numerals as the means of counting in every field of our life and work. Not only by the necessity required by our PC-s but likewise in view of the simplest problems we have to solve. Nevertheless, all the form systems of human speech tend to prove that man's consciousness of numeration took place in a period of development, in which languages (language groups and families) already possessed their solid and fixed grammatical and lexical systems having syntax and for the most part also morphology including a formal classification of word categories. But we do *not* know any language which would possess anyhow a separate word class of numerals like nouns or verbs etc. Numerals can in all these languages belong to (one or more) several word classes as to substantives (like *hundred*), to adjectives or adverbs (like *hundredfold*), to verbs (like *to double/ duplicate*). They constitute a particular "class" exclusively on the level of semantics.

The question is *what* way has led to the perception of numbering and counting? No language is known without any numeral system but these systems are extremely different in different languages. The lowest and most primitive stage is shown by languages with a simple binary: the speaker has a word for "one" and another for "two" denoting at the same time also "many" and "much". At the next stage of development binary turns out to be fixed and this "twofold" thinking makes possible to go on in counting in forms as $2 + 1 = 3, 2 + 2 = 4, 2 + 2 + 1 = 5$ etc. The basic pattern of such binaries is the reality surrounding humanity: we have – like many races of animals – two hands, feet, eyes, ears, nostrils, birds have two wings and so on. Some languages came thinking in binary up to the number 10 and what is more than 10 they simply call "many" or "much". Binary can be set forth to a fourfold system as by the Hoka-Indians in California: they have separate words for the numerals 1 till 4 and the rest of numerals they produce in a way of addition like $4 + 1 = 5$, $4 + 2 = 6$, or sometimes even by multiplication like $2 \times 4 = 8$ or combining both operations like $2 \times 4 + 1 = 9$. The background of this kind of counting is the reality of four fingers plus the thumb being apposable to the other fingers. The thumb is involved in the sextuple systems of some African languages with addition of the other hand as one more unity and from the number 6 on they operate likewise with additions and multiplications in the form $6 + 1 = 7$ or $6 \times 2 = 12$.

The first qualitative change developed in including other parts of the body, first of all, obviously, the hand = 5 fingers, 2 hands = 10 fingers, one foot = further 5 "fingers" (= toes), 2 feet = further 10 units, hands and feet totally 20 units. In this way it is also possible that several languages come up to several numeral systems. It is not an accident that many languages use the same word for "hand" and "five" like Samoan (*lima* "1. hand; 2. five"): in languages as Keva – New Guinea – with a finger counting without the thumb the word for "hand" means also 4, in this case *ki*) – or what is more – the same word for "twenty" and "man" (having 10 fingers and 10 toes, i.e. 20 units on hands and feet), so in the basic language of Hungarian (*húsz* "20" from Archaic *hú* "man") like the situation in Ono (Papuan) where the word group *nei mane korop* "the whole man" functions as the numeral for 20.

Decimal and vigesimal systems based upon the numbers 10 or 20 can also be combined and such intersections now and then produce curiosities like French *soixante-dix*, i.e. $60 + 10 = 70$ (NB: 60 is 3×20!), *quatre-vingt*, i.e. $4 \times 20 = 80$ and *quatre-vingt-dix*, i.e. $4 \times 20 + 10 = 90$. These French numerals are relics of a vigesimal system of Celtic or maybe older origin in a genuine decimal system of IE. languages. Something like this we find in Germanic too: Engl. *twenty* as well as Germ. *zwanzig* originally means 2×10. A crossing of a duodecimal and decimal system is evident in Engl. *eleven*, *twelve* and Germ. *elf*, *zwölf* which words consist of the elements *one-/ein-* or, *two-/zwei-* "2" and Old Engl. *-leofan*, Old Germ. *-lif*, literally "one or two left over ten". (The second part of these numerals is still living in Engl. *leave* and Germ. *bleiben*.) Accordingly, the Germanic word for 100, namely *hund*, meant "hundred and twenty".

Not only addition and multiplication can be used in forming numerals. Languages are known using subtraction for this purpose (too). In Ainu in Japan: $10 - 4 = 6$, $10 - 3 = 7$, etc. In Dravidian as well as in some Uralic languages we find forms like $10 - 2 = 8$. This reminds us of Lat. *duodeviginti* $= 20 - 2 = 18$, *undeviginti* $= 20 - 1 = 19$, even another evidence of primacy of the vigesimal system against our decimal system having the man as a whole as its mental base.

It must have been a thorny path that has led to our modern mathematical logic, and the numeral systems of human languages show a lot of prelogical relics in this curious evolution. Quite a curious and extreme way hereabout we see in the Papuan language Telefol. The speakers begin to count on the fingers of the left hand and set it forth over neck and head up and then down to the fingers of the right hand and can count 27 units, i.e. they have 27 numerals, every one of which they lexically identify with the names for the corresponding parts of the body:

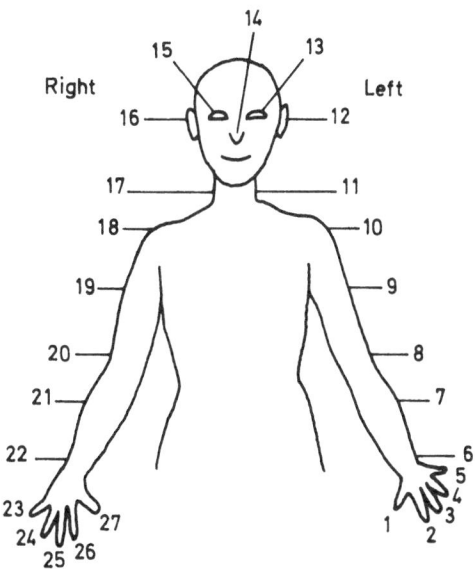

So it is no wonder that speakers of a language with so complicated systems switched over to simpler numeral systems of other languages. Chamorro speakers (Marianas Islands in the Pacific) use the Spanish counting system almost exclusively. The pre-Spanish system is no longer used and by about 1950 no one could remember it. Today the English (= American) system is being used more and more, particularly when counting money.

Correspondence: C. J. Hutterer, Department of Linguistics, Karl-Franzens-Universität, Universitätsplatz 3, A-8010 Graz, Austria.

Acta Neurochirurgica (1993) [Suppl] 56: 6–8

The Role of Music and Song in Human Communication

J. Ujfalussy

Institute of Musicology, Academy of Sciences, Budapest, Hungary

Summary

It is only on the higher level of abstraction and generalization that the two human branches of acoustic communication, speech and music are separated from each other.

Speech is primarily adjusted to the conceptual-verbal symbols and representation of an objectified, static world. In the linguistic communication the main role is played by the elements of noise, the consonants. It has never been doubted that music is a kind of communication, the mediator of human relationships, but it has been a question what music wants to express.

Since the Pythagoreans, some believe to find the key to interpreting its message in the commun quantifiable nature of the musical medium and the cosmos. Another historical tradition considered music as the direct expression of human emotions. Representants of the doctrine of imitation derived music from the intonation of speech and the text seems for many to be a support to "understand" music.

Music separated from the primary source of sound phenomena and their direct sensual effect constructed a specific communication system. It possesses an inestimable potential richness of discrete pitches and times, colours and sound intensity. The infinite potentials of successive and simultaneous combinations are suitable for erecting the audible, dynamic models of human relations and types of behaviour, internal events and interactions, different situations.

European polyphony established a strictly regulated, closed syntax of musical communication which comes close to conceptual precision. Its logic is based upon the natural potentials of the kinship of pitches and the human organ of hearing. The live, mobile network of the relations thus created is regulated by a further developed quasi-binary logic. The hidden sensual moment of musical sounding makes the message into an emotional, aesthetic experience. The balance and relationship of the logical and sensual moments are decisive from the point of view of the artistic-aesthetic value of music.

The typical situations of everyday life are coupled with the appropriate ways of musical expressions, born together with them as tunes, sound sequences, rhythms, signals, suitable musical instruments, etc. They are identified with the situations and gain the same meaning.

All sounds and noises carry and convey information at least pertaining to their living or lifeless sources, their position, movement, quantitative and qualitative characteristics to intellects which are able to perceive acoustic impulses, compare them with those known to them as well as identify them. Under common living circumstances, communication systems in the actual sense come into being in populations where regulated relationships develop between the members of the community on the one hand and between them and their environment on the other, where emission and reception, communication and perception function mutually.

Ethology is familiar with the different acoustic communication systems of the world of animals. In accordance with the two large human systems, they are referred to either as language or as music, especially in the case of birds. A number of human communities use a mixture of means of expressions which may at times be qualified as speech and at times as music. Let us think of the African drum languages or a record from the phonogramme collection of Erich von Hornbostel. In it a young man from Cameroon conveys the news that "A woman has born many children but now no longer has a child" by speaking, drumming, singing and whistling[1].

The promiscuity of the acoustic means of communication correlates with the complexity of the different human relationships as they permeate each other in a non-differentiated unity and live together in everyday life. Here the reactions, viewpoints of the objective moment and the participants, the communicator and the recipient are two aspects of the same situation and its audible communication. It is only on the higher level of abstraction and generalization that the two

---

[1] Example 1. Demonstration Collection of E. M. von Hornbostel and the Berlin Phonogramm Archiv. Indiana 1962. Indiana University, Ethnic Folkways Library 4175. Demonstrations Sammlung Nr. 82. (Ankermann, Kamerun 1909) Disc II, Side B, Band 3

human branches of acoustic communication, speech and music are separated from each other.

Speech is primarily adjusted to the conceptual-verbal symbols and representation of an objectified, static world. In the linguistic communication the main role is played by the elements of noise, the consonants. Conceptual understanding, the meaning of the acoustic system of symbols is based upon them. For example, the writing of the Semitic languages – as well as stenography – indicate the consonants.

Music is developed overwhelmingly from "vocal" elements. As a kind of art, it increasingly gives up the primary, tactile representation and depiction of the individual objective phenomena. Its way of communication differs from the usual one, and its meaning is qualified as dubious, intangible, mysterious by practical thinking, and serves as an interaction with supernatural powers as a medium of communication in the animistic rituals. The well-known "drug effect" of music also participates in this function. The specific formation of sounds of the East-Asian peoples, "flat" singing, which may be observed in the Hungarian peasant singing as well, originates not from the inborn, organic characteristics of their articulation basis but from sacral, ritual tradition[2].

André Schaeffner points to the magic origin of singing, the effects of tone and noise of the singing of different peoples, which are so very different from the image of European singing, the so-called "natural" way of singing. Schaeffner refers to Kurt Sachs whose opinion was that our "natural" ideal of singing hardly goes back farther in history than the Renaissance. In this Sachs discovered the sign of singing having been subject to a process of laicisation[3].

Now we hear the song of a Mongolian shaman. The ritual starts with a usual pentatonic tune. During the repetitions it loses its continuous, structured form and only fragments of it remain. They are similar to animal cries[4].

It has never been doubted that music is a kind of communication, the mediator of human relationships, but it has been a question of debate what music wants to express. People either try to find tactile, objective points, pictorial world which they believe to recognize in other arts. And if they fail to find such phenomena in music, they look upon it as a direct form of appearance of quite general laws of nature. Since the Pythagoreans, some believe to find the key to interpreting and explaining its message in the common quantifiable nature of the musical medium and the cosmos. For Leibniz music was "excertitium arithmetices occultum nescientis se animi", "the secret arithmetic exercise of the unconscious soul"[5].

Another historical tradition considered music as the direct expression of human emotions. It was inclined to identify mechanically certain musical patterns with the appropriate emotional manifestations. This approach, the doctrine of affections characterized a great era of European music interpretations.

Its close relative is the doctrine of imitations, a misunderstood development of the concept of Aristotle related to imitation in the Modern Age. Its representatives, including Diderot, derived music from the intonation of speech. They looked upon speech as the living pattern of musical imitation. In the meantime the text has seemed for many to be a support which makes music understandable up to the present day. This illusion and the development of the cultures of mother language-literature have strengthened the views related to the priority of speech and vocal music with lyric since Plato. They are not supported by the facts of historical development.

In opposition, it is just the task of music to demonstrate that arts which apparently introduce the objective face of the world use the objective elements of their environment as a medium only. The individual objective moments obtain a new, specific function only valid in the system of the whole of the work.

As music became separated from the primary source of sound phenomena, their colour and noise characteristics and direct sensual effect, it constructed a specific communication system. In it direct sensuality feeds the actual artistic message as an emotional fuel. Music possesses an inestimable potential richness of discrete pitches and times, colours and sound intensity. The infinite potentials of successive and simultaneous combinations are suitable for creating the audible, dynamic models of human relations and types of behaviour, internal events and interactions, different situations. This nature of music hides its kinship with mathe-

[2] Example 2. Hungarian Folk Music 1. Disc II B 12. (G. Paulovics, Fedemes, Heves-m. 1966)

[3] Andre Schaeffner (1936) Origine des Instruments de Musique, Payot, Paris, p 15, note 2

[4] Example 3. Dahat Shaman Song, raising of spirits. Collection of the Institute of Musicology of the Hungarian Academy of Sciences. (V. Dioszegi, Mongolia, 1966, No 51)

[5] G. W. Leibniz. Epistolae, ed. Korholt Leibzig. Epistola CLIV ad Chr. Goldbachium, 17, 04, 1712, pp 240–241. Quoted by Dr. Hermann Pfrogner (1954) Musik. Geschichte ihrer Deutung. Munchen, K. A. Freiburg, p 191

matics mentioned frequently and not the quantitative measurability of their media. An important role in this creative process is played by gestures. This is unduly neglected by European thinking which is characterized by its rather verbal-conceptual nature. It is sufficient to refer to the different dances and their participation in music semantics. By the way, speech is a kind of intensive, audible system of gestures.

European polyphony established a strictly regulated, closed syntax of musical communication which comes close to conceptual precision, making possible the creation of great instrumental works. Its logic is based upon the natural potentials of the kinship of pitches and the human organ of hearing. The pitch relationships fit into a certain hierarchy. The live, mobile network of the relations thus created is regulated by a further developed, quasi-binary logic. At the same time this network constitutes a virtual quasi-space as well. In it the pitch relationships are compared to each other along a vertical axis, like the steps of a ladder. The hidden sensual moment of musical sounding makes the message into an emotional, aesthetic experience with its tone and noise elements and dynamism. The balance and relationship of the logical and sensual moments are decisive from the point of view of the artistic-aesthetic value of music.

The typical situations of everyday life are coupled with the appropriate ways of musical expression, born together with them as tunes, sound sequences, rhythms, signals, suitable musical instruments, etc. They are identified with the situations and gain the same meaning. They are evoked in the great musical works too, becoming parts of the identity consciousness of communities. Thus, for example, the music of the bagpipes – mostly in F major – means the village in Viennese classics.

In the last movement of Beethoven's 9th Symphony, after an intense crescendo, a long fermata, we hear quite soft beats of drums. A new version of the known theme is heard, a march. It is accompanied by percussion[6].

What does this musical situation express? The theme itself is connected to the melodious phraseology of the French Revolution. This is conspicuously demonstrated by a line of the Carmagnole. In those days the specific instrumentation, the rich accompaniment by percussion was referred to as "türkische Musik". The noble Turks and Persians were favourite figures of the literature of the Age of Enlightenment. They were the representatives of elevated, human thinking in opposition to the biased, conservative Europeans. That is why the embraced millions of the East are approaching with "Turkish music" in Beethoven's vision to participate with full rights in the great, joint celebration of liberated mankind. This circle of connotations is conjured up by the Turkish version of the revolutionary theme.

This degree of musical "message" is characteristic of a highly diverse and differentiated society. This is the world of multinational music industry, telecommunication, mass media. Here the loud, audible reaction to the artistic message on the part of the audience does not materialize. It experiences and internalizes the message in silence, at best reacts to it by applause. The function of music to convey a message seems to be one-sided again, and it really is one-sided not infrequently. In his "Aesthetics" Nicolai Hartmann analyzed the layers of the musical work[7], and they are the layers of reception at the same time too. To investigate which groups of the real and potential audience reach which layers of the different musical works, or how music as communication lives and exerts its influence in society, is the difficult task of music sociology.

Correspondence: J. Ujfalussy, Institute of Musicology, Academy of Sciences, V. Nádor u. 7, H-1361, Budapest, Hungary.

---

[6] Example 4. Beethoven. Symphony No 9. Finale, Allegro assai vivace. Alla Marcia

[7] Nicolai Hartmann. Ästhetik. Berlin, 1953, de Gruyter, pp 197–212

Acta Neurochirurgica (1993) [Suppl] 56: 9–13

Communication in Animals

G. Ádám

Department of Comparative Physiology, Eötvös Loránd University, Budapest, Hungary

Summary

The paper deals with the antecedents of human speech in animals, more precisely with the problems of continuity versus discontinuity in communication between the different species of vertebrates. It puts emphasis on higher classes of mammals, namely monkeys and apes. Three ancient structures and mechanisms are listed which may have a role as forerunners of the development of human speech: (1) the activity of the mimic muscles of the cheeks and of the jaws, (2) the evolution of sound-producing specialized membranes in the laryngeal respiratory passages, and (3) the development of hemispheric asymmetries of the brain, which culminated in the emergence of the specific speech areas of the dominant hemisphere in humans.

The history of the research of animal language cannot avoid the survey of the fascinating trials made on anthropoid apes. The paper briefly summarizes the four approaches (American Sign Language, plastic tokens, keyboard systems and mimics) with the conclusion that continuity can be demonstrated in brain lateralization and in cognitive abilities, but a marked discontinuity between animal communication and human speech is evident.

The main object of this Convention, human communication and speech, cannot be completely explored without the treatment of its history in the evolution of *homo sapiens*. In other words it was a proper decision of the organizers of this meeting to include communication in animals among the main topics. As I have taught Comparative Physiology for many years at the University of Budapest, I must deal with this subject every year evoking discussions and debates among my students.

My presentation will deal with the antecedents of human speech in animals, more precisely with the problems of continuity versus discontinuity in oral communication between the different species of higher classes of vertebrates, including man. The sequence of the following ideas and data presumes a certain degree of inevitable anthropomorphism in the description of verbal behaviour. It endows an animal with psychological and behavioural traits like those of humans and supposes that it acts from similar motives. General and specific anthropomorphism are both included in our scientific reasoning. General man-centred biological thought refers to the endowment of a general purposefulness to higher animals, whereas specific anthropomorphism deals "only" with special mental and behavioural states, like our topic, the communicative behaviour.

The main issue of this paper can be outlined as follows: whether communication in higher vertebrates on the one hand and human language on the other can be regarded as governed by laws of *continuity or* whether *discontinuity* is characteristic in their evolution? I will try to give an approximate answer to this question, taking into account merely the vertebrate world, although it is common knowledge that communication between individuals practically exists in all known species.

No doubt that among the four main modalities of physical signals, namely optical, auditive, tactile and chemical, the latter must historically have been the very first. Chemical signal systems, the main transmission mechanisms among nerve cells in a multicellular organism were used and are still utilized as channels of information between organisms. The summit of chemical communication is reached by insects, which employ a very rich variety of alarm and attractive substances. Common knowledge that all vertebrate species make use of it, although sight, sound and touch prevail in later development.

By definition an animal is considered to have communicated with another animal when it can be shown to have influenced, or rather to have manipulated its behaviour through specific signals. Either of the above-mentioned four qualities of signals must be specific, namely species-specific and/or individual-specific and finally message-specific. This latter quality indicates that *it has meaning*, in other words it carries information. Ethology claims that the genes of both the sender and the receiver of the information will benefit by communication. But in analyzing this ethological dogma one must be very careful, since in the course of natural selection no two animals have, strictly speaking, the same genetic interests! Consequently, in the course of evolution, signals must be regarded as specific tools by which animals manipulate the behaviour of competitors in order to benefit from the genomes of the signaller, sometimes even at the cost of the receiver.

I must emphasize again the message-specificity of signals between two animals, since these signals will alter the behaviour of the receiver animal, if it bears information. A message, in order to be informative, must be to some extent somewhat new to the receiver; this feature of novelty enables one to define it mathematically. In this respect most of the inter-animal messages carry information, since these signals reduce the prior uncertainty caused by other signals. Prior uncertainty is measurable in terms of probabilities. If the message enables the receiver to come to a decision between two alternatives which had previously been equally probable, say the approach of a predator or of a prey animal, then one bit of information has been disclosed. Thus one bit is defined as the quantity of information needed to halve the receiver's prior uncertainty, to enable him to make a decision between two alternatives which were equally probable. The ecology of animal communication is able, consequently, to measure and to quantify the messages between individuals within, or between the species. The quantification of animal messages might be useful and practical, but many ecologists think that the qualitative rather than the quantitative aspect of signals is appropriate. Consequently, I will not make use of this binary system of information when shortly dealing with some cardinal aspects of the evolution of animal communication.

In the world of invertebrates transmission of information is universal. Chemical, auditory and visual signals are equally widespread, e.g. *ants* use alarm substances to alert the colony in case of danger. The female *silk moth* attracts the male by secreting the well known Bombykol. Auditory signals are used by a very great number of insects, the record is probably held by the *mole cricket*. This tiny animal emits acoustical signals which can be detected a half kilometre away. The visual information transmitted by the *honey-bee* has been thoroughly analysed. The round dance and the waggle dance of this rather simple creature informs the rest of the colony of the distance and the direction of the food,

using the sun as a reference point. It is considered that the bee dance is a rather special case, a rare exception in which the meaning of the animal signal is better thought of as referring to external cues. More usually the message reflects the internal motivational state of the signaller. This latter is the case in all vertebrate species.

The world of lower and higher vertebrates has been extensively studied from the point of view of communication. The modern forerunner was undoubtedly Charles Darwin[5], who in his book "The Expression of the Emotions in Man and Animals" published in 1872 has shown that animal signals have evolved from non-signal movements, which originally served useful day-to-day purposes. The denomination of *ritualization* has been given to the evolution of signals from non-signals. Many birds communicate by means of feather-erection behaviour, which originally served thermoregulation. In general, some incomplete intention movements are the most probable antecedents for ritualization. A dog baring its teeth by drawing back the lips – displaying a signal of threat – is a good example of such a movement (which, by the way, can be regarded as the ancestor of the human smile and grimace). According to many researchers, emotionally induced exaggerated breathing movements may have been the starting actions of today's bird song and sound signalling of mammals: the mammalian pharynx and the bird's syrinx have evolved from the upper respiratory tracts of these groups of animals.

The main question at issue in the present paper can be outlined in the form of enumerating the candidates which presumably may have a role as antecedents of the development of human speech in the ritual and non-ritual communicative signals of vertebrate animals. *Three such ancient structures and mechanisms* can be listed.

First: the development and the activity of the mimic muscles of the cheeks and of the jaws, mentioned above;

Second: the development of sound-producing specialized membranes in the laryngeal respiratory passages, culminating in the appearance of mammalian vocal cords;

Third: the evolution of hemispheric asymmetries of the brain, which culminated in the emergence of the specific speech areas in the dominant hemisphere of humans.

I will not come back to the first function. The main ideas of Darwin still prevail in our contemporary conception of the relation of animal and human face musculature.

As far as the second problem is concerned, Lev Vygotski[17], in the middle of the thirties had published his principle according to which the parallel developments of animal cognition and sound-emitting apparatus could not result in the emergence of verbalization mechanisms in higher mammals – not even in apes – since these two lines of evolution could never meet. This is in contrast to human development, in course of which the evolution of cognition and that of the anatomy of the laryngeal and buccal structures met each other a few million years ago.

The third ancient mechanism is the most intriguing and controversial: asymmetries in species other than man are widespread, but it is far from being proved that these shifts to the right or to the left in the animal kingdom are in relation to the development of human brain lateralization. First of all it must be emphasized that the prevailing tendency toward lateralization, namely toward dextrality is almost unique in humans, but from an individual aspect many other species display right-left asymmetries, although their direction may not be regular between individuals.

Asymmetries among invertebrates are common. Enough to mention the "clawedness" of crabs: in certain species the left claw is consistently larger, while in other species it is the right. The lungs of certain species of snakes are asymmetrical, and genital asymmetries in insects are common. Most of the gastropod species show a highly consistent tendency in the direction of shell coiling, etc. It would be a bold, although a risky and unjustified proposition to relate these invertebrate asymmetries with human brain lateralization.

As far as asymmetries in vertebrates are concerned, the habenular nucleus of the brain is frequently larger on one side for most species of lower vertebrates (fishes, amphibians) linked to lateralization in locomotion. The song organ in birds, the syrinx, is always asymmetrical, the nervous control is ipsilateral. That means that loss of song is irreversible if left-sided damage occurs in the adult male canary, but in young birds the right side can take over. Some other complex behaviour in birds is known to be lateralized, like discrimination learning, imprinting, habituation, etc. as shown by Nottebohm.

The most intensive studies in brain asymmetries in animals have been undertaken in mammals. Denenberg[6] et al. reported that handling and environmental enrichment affected the right hemisphere more than the left in young rats. The cortical thickness of the right hemisphere is greater than that of the left particularly in male animals, which show also the prevalence of the right brain in emotionality, agression, etc. An innate lateralization of handedness is also demonstrated in rodents linked probably to the slight asymmetry in the availability of catecholamines in the extrapyramidal motor nuclei (e.g. the nigro-striatal nuclei).

In monkeys the lateralization of handedness effects are similar to those in rodents, being strongly affected by experience and practice. That means that it can be reversed by conditional reinforcement, which suggests that this function is not homologous to that in humans. In split-brain monkeys either hemisphere can equally learn visual discrimination. However, some evidence proves the left lateralization of nonvocal auditory function in the macaque monkey. Dewson has demonstrated that pure tone versus noise signal discrimination is impaired after a lesion to the left, but not to the right auditory cortex.

The studies of brain asymmetries in apes evoked and still evokes the most vivid interest among researchers in that field, since it might have immediate relation to human brain lateralization and speech. Almost a century ago Cunningham (1892)[4] already alluded to brain asymmetries in chimpanzee, orangutan and baboon brains. Le May and Geschwind (1975)[12] demonstrated that the point of termination of the Sylvian fissure was higher on the right side than on the left in the orangutan, chimpanzee and gorilla. Yeni-Komshian (1976)[18] found that the Sylvian fissure was longer on the left side. Cain and Wada (1979)[1] showed larger frontal lobes in the right hemispheres in baboons than in humans. Do these findings indicate that these subhuman species are apt to generate speech, i.e. to form novel propositions? The answer – as we will make clear soon – is probably negative. Apes are, in all probability, not using those areas of the brain that correspond to the human speech areas, that is the parts in the vicinity of the temporal auditory cortex (Wernicke's area) and areas near the facial motor cortex in the frontal lobe (Broca's area). At the very most the available data suggest that subhuman primates are perhaps preadapted for the evolution of lateralized speech systems.

The history of the research of animal thought and animal language has been and is actually still the story of famous anthropoid apes. From the findings of Köhler in the thirties up to the present, the scientific community as well as the broader public knows these apes by name, since they displayed the amazing performance of animal cognition, reasoning and other mental qualities. But what about the acquisition of human language?

It is common knowledge that apes display a remarkable lack of interest in imitating human speech. The gorilla and the orang-utang are fairly quiet species, the chimpanzee is a little bit more vocal and more social. No wonder that human language teaching experiments have been undertaken mostly on individuals of this species, although the social vocabulary of these animals in their natural environment is very, very, poor! Comparative anatomists often emphasize that the sound-producing apparatus of these apes is physically inadequate for emitting human speech. The construction of the vocal cords of the larynx, the resonating cavities of the throat and mouth and the adjusting mechanisms of lips and tongue are all incapable of articulation. The first domesticated ape explored scientifically, the gorilla John Daniel of Cunningham who behaved himself excellently in human company, could not emit words at all. The Kelloggs reported a similar unsuccessful trial with their infant chimpanzee in the early twenties. The Hayes couple, two decades later, succeeded in teaching their animal, Vicki to pronounce four words (Mama, Poppa, cup and up).

This initial failure inspired and forced their followers to try different approaches. As we all know, *four* diverse techniques were undertaken. The first of these was begun by the Gardners who taught some 160 words of the American Sign Language to the female chimpanzee *Washoe*. The next famous case of the same approach was reported by Terrace who trained the male chimpanzee Nim Chimpsky to emit whole sentences. Subsequently the success of these workers has been confirmed by other systematic studies.

The *second* approach used coloured plastic symbols as words. Premack developed this training system and taught his chimpanzee Sarah to learn a vocabulary of 130 words. The plastic tokens used did not physically resemble the object they referred to. Sarah, one of four apes trained by Premack, could form rather sophisticated short sentences, although this achievement cannot be regarded as the use of any kind of grammar nor to call it true syntax.

The *third* training method consisted of an automated keyboard system operated by the female chimpanzee Lana trained by Rumbaugh. It has been proved that the chimpanzees can make a wide range of requests for desired objects, can name objects and events, and even can communicate with their trainers and other chimpanzees. Lana was even able to label labels rather than only label objects: for instance if shown the pattern "banana" she could press the key meaning "food".

The *fourth* approach used limb movements, gazing directions and face muscle responses reinforcing the above findings.

What general rules can be summarized from all these very, very, attractive and intriguing ape experiments? Do these trials prove the possibility of teaching animals human language, or at least a rudimentary human speech? I believe the answer is absolutely negative. The gorillas, the orangutans and the chimpanzees are highly developed species of animals, with sophisticated cognitive structures, but language is another story. One must remember that the analogies between the demonstrated performances of chimpanzees and the human use of speech are extremely doubtful! As many sceptic opinions emphasize, the acquisition of the described abilities can be explained by high cognitive performances and by surreptitious, covert sensory skills of these primates in the course of well known classical and/or operant conditioning. I must repeatedly mention Vygotski's principle: apes are champions in cognition, but inferior in communication!

Consequently continuity can be demonstrated in brain morphology and lateralization, as well as in the development of cognitive abilities, but a marked discontinuity can be stated between animal communication and human speech.

Finally, let me quote Noam Chomsky: "Can we expect to find, in other organisms, faculties closely analogous to the human language capacity? It is conceivable, but not very likely. That would constitute a kind of biological miracle, rather similar to the discovery, on some unexplored island, of a species of bird that had never thought to fly until instructed to do so through human intervention. Language must surely confer enormous selectional advantage. It is difficult to imagine that some other species, say the chimpanzee, has the capacity for language but has never thought to put it to use. Nor is there any evidence that this biological miracle has occurred. On the contrary, the interesting investigations of the capacity of the higher apes to acquire symbolic systems seem to me to support the traditional belief that even the most rudimentary properties of language lie well beyond the capacities of an otherwise intelligent ape".

References

1. Cain DP, Wada JA (1979) An anatomical asymmetry in the baboon brain. Brain Behav Evol 16: 222–226
2. Chomsky N (1980) Rules and representations. Columbia University Press, New York
3. Cunningham A (1921) A gorilla's life in civilization. Bulletin of the Zoological Societies, New York, Vol 24, pp 118
4. Cunningham DF (1892) Contribution to the surface anatomy of the cerebral hemispheres. Royal Irish Academy, Dublin, p 167

5. Darwin C (1965) The expression of the emotions in man and animals. University of Chicago Press

6. Denenberg VH (1981) Hemispheric laterality in animals and the effects of early experience. Behavioural and Brain Sciences 4: 1–49

7. Dewson JH (1977) Preliminary evidence of hemispheric asymmetry of auditory function in monkeys. In: Harnad S, Doty RW, Jaynes J, Goldstein C, Krauthamer K (eds) Lateralization in the nervous system. Academic Press, New York, pp 63–71

8. Gardner RA, Gardner BT (1969) Teaching sign language to a chimpanzee. Science 165: 664–672

9. Hayes KJ, Hayes C (1952) Imitation in a home raised chimpanzee. J Comp Physiol Psychol 46: 470–474

10. Kellogg WN (1968) Communication and language in the home-raised chimpanzee. Science 162: 423–427

11. Kohler W (1929) Gestalt Psychology. Liveright, New York

12. Le May M, Gechwind N (1975) Hemispheric differences in the brains of great apes. Brain Behav Evol 11: 48–52

13. Nottebohm F (1979) Origins and mechanisms in the establishment of cerebral dominance. In: Gazzaniga MS (ed) Handbook of behavioural neurology, Neuropsychology, Vol 2. Plenum, New York, pp 295–344

14. Premack D (1976) Intelligence in ape and man. Lawrence Erlbaum, Hillsdale

15. Rumbaugh D (ed) (1977) Language learning by a chimpanzee: The LANA Project. Academic Press, New York

16. Terrace HS (1980) Nim. Eyre Methuen, London

17. Vygotsky LS (1962) Thought and language. MIT Press, Cambridge, Mass

18. Yeni-Komshian G, Benson D (1976) Anatomical study of cerebral asymmetry in the temporal lobe of humans, chimpanzees and rhesus monkeys. Science 192: 387–389

Correspondence: G. Ádám, Department of Comparative Physiology, Eötvös Lóránd University, Muzeum Körut 4-A, H-1088, Budapest, Hungary.

Acta Neurochirurgica (1993) [Suppl] 56: 14–16

Language Families

Á. Nádasdy

Department of English, Eötvös Lóránd University, Budapest, Hungary

Summary

The "genetic" relatedness of languages and their grouping into "families" is a metaphor taken from biology. The family tree model fails to account for the mutual influence of languages; hence the "wave" theory. Family relationships are set up by systematically recurring phonetic differences, rather than similarities. The 4,000 languages are grouped in about 50 language families: linguistics tries to find their common features, called "language universals".

Introduction

A language family is a group of languages which are genetically related to each other, but not to any language outside the family; thus a language family is the largest possible group of related (i.e. cognate) languages. This of course is a heavily biological metaphor – like so much in historical and comparative linguistics, it comes from the first half of the 19th century, and was influenced by evolutionism, Darwinism, or "Naturgeschichte", as the German word aptly describes it. Just like animals were classified into families (e.g. the cat family), so were languages – except that in zoology families are further grouped into larger units of order, class, and phylum. In linguistics, however, we normally have to stop at the family level, for reasons that we shall deal with below.

The number of languages spoken in the world can be estimated to be somewhere between three and five thousand. The uncertainty of the guess is caused by the fact that there still may be languages spoken in remote places that we do not know about, but also by the difficulty of distinguishing between language and dialect: often it is just cultural or political tradition that labels two closely related dialects as different languages (as in the case of, say, Hindi and Urdu, or Czech and Slovak), while the opposite may also happen, i.e. two widely divergent idioms, which would warrant being called separate languages, are nevertheless traditionally label-led as merely dialects of one and the same language (as in the case of Chinese or German). The languages of the world are now usually grouped into about 50 families, which would give an average of about 80 languages per family.

Table 1. *The World's Language Families* (with main branches)

Indo-European
  Germanic, Italic-Romance, Celtic, Hellenic, Albanian, Slavic, Baltic, Armenian, Hittite, Indo-Iranian.
Uralic
  Finno-Ugric (e.g. Finnish, Hungarian), Samoyed.
Altaic
  Turkic, Mongolian, Manchu-Tungusic.
Caucasian (e.g. Georgian)
Basque
Dravidian (e.g. Tamil, Telugu, Malayalam)
Sino-Tibetan
  Chinese, Tibeto-Burman, Thai, Miao-Yao.
Japanese
Korean
Ainu
Mon-Khmer (e.g. Cambodian)
Vietnamese
Malayo-Polynesian (e.g. Indonesian, Maori, Hawaiian)
Papuan
Australian (Aboriginal)
Paleo-Asiatic or Paleo-Siberian
  (e.g. Chukchee, Kamchadal, Yukagir).
Eskimo-Aleut
Hamito-Semitic
  Semitic (e.g. Arabic, Herbrew, Amharic), Berber (e.g. Tuareg), Cushitic (e.g. Somali), Egyptian (e.g. Coptic), Chadic (e.g. Hausa).
Niger-Congo
  Western Sudanic (e.g. Ibo), Benue-Congo, including Bantu (e.g. Swahili, Zulu, Xhosa).
Chari-Nile
  Sudanic (e.g. Nubian).
Khoisan (e.g. Bushman, Hottentot)
+ about 5 further families in Africa

North American Indian: about 20 families.
South American Indian: 3 large families?

Altogether about 50 families for the world's ca 4000 languages.

In actual fact some families consist of one language only – which is an elegant way of saying that we are unable to classify them with any other family (e.g. Basque or Japanese) – and, at the other end of the scale, there are families with several hundred languages in them, like Indo-European or Niger-Congo. A fairly comprehensive list of the language families of the Old World can be seen in Table 1.

Establishing Family Membership

On what grounds does the linguist put a language into one family or another (or into none)? We said above that family members must be "genetically related". Now this is again a biological metaphor, since obviously languages are not made of living matter to have genetic relationships. What we mean by genetically related (or cognate) is that the two languages are divergent developments of the same earlier language: in other words, that some time ago they used to be the same language, and an unbroken line of successive speech communities has been using them, introducing different innovations that have led to their divergences.

This implies two things. One, that borrowed material (i.e. loan-words from one language into another) does not constitute proof for relatedness. The Hungarian sentence under Example 1 has been constructed almost entirely of words of Latin origin, but this does not prove that the two languages are related – borrowing is a social, cultural, or political phenomenon, i.e. it is due to extralinguistic factors.

Example 1. A krónikus bronchitisz urbanizációs probléma.

As can be seen, similarity is open to suspicion because it may be due to borrowing, or – on a small scale – to mere chance. Therefore the linguist looks for better proof, and finds it in differences which are regular. If language A always has sound x in some position where language B has sound y, this is good ground for supposing a genetic relationship. Such a correspondence is called a "sound law" and shows that one (or both) languages introduced an innovation at some point. Look at the Hungarian and Finnish examples in Table 2.

Thus we can establish that Hungarian *ház* "house" is related to Finnish *kota* "hut" – even though it might have seemed that it was related to the German *Haus*, which is more similar both in meaning and form!

Family Relationships

If we compare several languages and find them to be related through such regular differences (the bigger the differences, the better, for the danger of dealing with borrowed material diminishes), we model their derivation on what is called a family tree. An example can be seen in Table 3.

The lines represent shared innovations (that is, changes away from the older form) which are shown by all the languages under the scope of that line. Thus for example, the line leading from Germanic to West Germanic represents some innovations shared by all the languages under it, but not by the others, the North and East Germanic languages.

There are problems with the family tree model, however. One is that you can often draw the lines in different ways, producing different subgroups – depending on what innovation you consider more important. Some authors, for example, group the West Germanic languages into English on the one hand and Dutch-German on the other, giving precedence to features shared by Dutch and German vis-á-vis English (and certainly they have many features in common that

Table 2. *Comparative Analysis*

Hungarian	Finnish	
ház	kota	"house; hut"
hó	kuu	"month"
hal	kala	"fish"
kő	kivi	"stone"
kéz	käsi	"hand"
kigyó	kyy	"snake"
száz	sata	"100"
vezet	vetää	"lead; pull"

Table 3. *Part of a Typical Family Tree* (simplified)

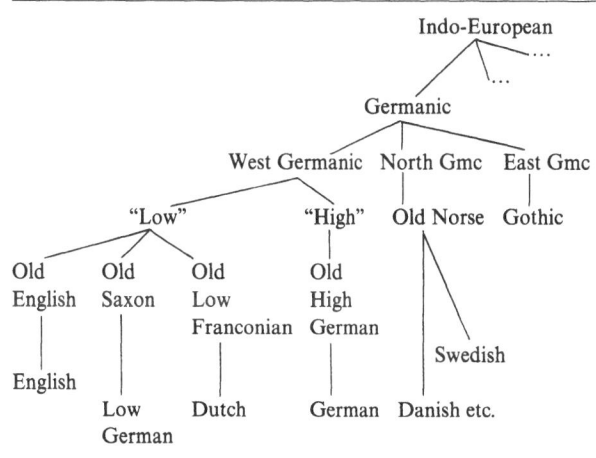

English lacks). That is to say, it is often fairly arbitrary what we consider as the decisive innovation.

The bigger problem with the family tree, however, concerns the very heart of the matter: the biological metaphor itself. Living beings, once they are born, remain genetically the same and do not influence the genetic makeup of their sisters or that of further offspring. Not so with languages: they often influence each other, and in ways that are more basic than borrowing. This is accounted for by the "wave" theory, which says that innovations may spread across an area like waves, irrespective of whether the languages spoken there are closely related or related at all. The result is a "linguistic area", which often cuts across linguistic families. A case in point is the monosyllabic nature of many South East Asian languages (Chinese, Vietnamese, Cambodian) which are otherwise genetically unrelated, i.e. show no regular correspondence or "sound laws". Whether such convergence can ultimately lead to a more or less unified language is an interesting question – there is nothing to exclude this, anyway. It is quite possible, then, that what is now a language family, i.e. a group of languages stemming from a common ancestor, had this common ancestor once produced by the areal convergence of several languages! After all, human speech is about a million years old, and we have records for only the last six thousand years; and, needless to say, even for those six thousand years we have ridiculously little evidence of what people spoke around the world.

Because languages may converge and diverge, and populations may even abandon their original language and adopt a new one (for example, that of the conquerors), we must be careful not to identify language with ethnicity. Obviously, the fact that American Negroes speak an Indo-European language says nothing about their ethnic background; such situations keep recurring in history and may blur the correspondence between race and language. Hungarian is related to Finnish; this leads many people to believe that the Hungarians are related to the Finns – an assumption that is contradicted by many other findings, such as archeology, music, religious history and others. Certainly the "default" proposition is that if the languages are related, the peoples are probably related too – but it may or may not be true.

A family, we said, is the largest group for which genetic relationship can be proved. And between families? This is a vexed question, for often there is evidence of links between families, but the material is simply not enough, or is not conclusive enough to say anything with reliability. Especially the families of Northern and Western Eurasia – Indo-European, Hamito-Semitic, Uralic, Altaic, and Paleo-Asiatic, offer correspondences that are stronger than mere chance would allow, yet they are still too weak to warrant anything but intelligent guesswork. Some scholars hope to find further evidence for such a "Nostratic" proto-family, but I am very sceptical.

Linguists are convinced that all languages are basically the same, since they are the product of the same human brain. We assume that there must be linguistic universals informing the system of each language – but we know fairly little about these as yet. We are faced with a bewildering variety on the surface, and it seems that all languages are constantly changing, converging, diverging, and so on. What we are trying to find out is what remains constant in them. The Classical Greek comedy writer Aristophanes has sheep on the stage and they say baa-baa. 2500 years later sheep still say the same; their "speech" is genetically coded. Obviously with humans the surface structure of language is not genetically coded, and is thus free to change – within certain limits. These are the limits that are probably genetically coded and constitute what can be called "human language".

References

1. Anttila R (1972) An introduction to historical and comparative linguistics. New York
2. Bynon T (1977/1983) Historical linguistics. Cambridge University Press
3. Katzner K (1977/1986) The languages of the world. Routledge, London
4. Meillet A, Cohen M (1952) Les langages du monde. Paris

Correspondence: Á. Nádasdy, Department of English, Eötvös Lóránd University, Muzeum körut 4-A, H-1088, Budapest, Hungary.

Acta Neurochirurgica (1993) [Suppl] 56: 17–19

Functional Anatomy of Human Speech

J. Szentágothai

Institute of Anatomy, Semmelweiss University, Budapest, Hungary

Summary

The outlines of an investigation into side differences between the *Planum temporale* (The Geschwind-Levitzky areas) of ten human brains are given. Volume of this area and cell numbers are clearly asymmetric, the left side being consequently larger by 38–34% over the same area at right. Cell density (cell No/volume) is virtually the same on both sides. Some comments upon the data are being made.

1. The Asymmetry of the Speech Areas

The title of this contribution may seem somewhat strange, so that it may need some explanation. To deal with and to ponder about the functional anatomy of such large areas of the brain, as those that have been identified as being involved – one way or another – with speech disorders (the classical speech areas: *Broca*'s area, the *Wernicke* area) do not offer any clue for comparison of the two sides of the brain. It is quite hopeless to think of any anatomical method that would enable us to compare possible asymmetries with any degree of confidence.

Fortunately, there is one relatively limited area of the temporal lobe: the region of the transverse gyri on the upper surface of the temporal lobe; the so-called *Planum temporale* or otherwise the surface hidden in the depth of the Sylvian fissure (in the classical literature Heschl's gyri [Heschl I. in front and Heschl II. to the rear]). In recent years this region has become important from a brief study by Geschwind and Levitsky in Science (1968)[1]. The crucial illustration of this study is being reproduced here in Fig. 1. The size difference of left over right is clearly visible, however, what is much more important, the restricted region indicated as *PT* (Planum temporale) is sufficiently restricted in size and its borders sufficiently marked to make it possible to make comparisons between relatively well-defined cortical regions of both hemispheres.

The results shown in Table 1 were – I should confess – a great disappointment. My expectation, on the basis of a general phylogenetic tendency – especially in the cerebral cortex – of a decrease in cell density: i.e. the phylogenetic development of the central organs is reflected much less in the increase of cell numbers, than in that of interneuron connexions (= the neuropil). So I expected that the development of a special genetically preprogrammed neural apparatus for speech would be reflected in an increase of the neuropil (non-cell tissue matter) on the left side, and not in an increase in cell numbers. The results show quite unequivocally that the *Planum temporale* contains 40 million more cells on the left side than on the right. There is, of course, no justification for arguing with facts. The facts show unequivocally – which corresponds also to the observations of Witelson and Pallie (1975)[2] about size differences left over right of the Planum temporale in the human newborn – that

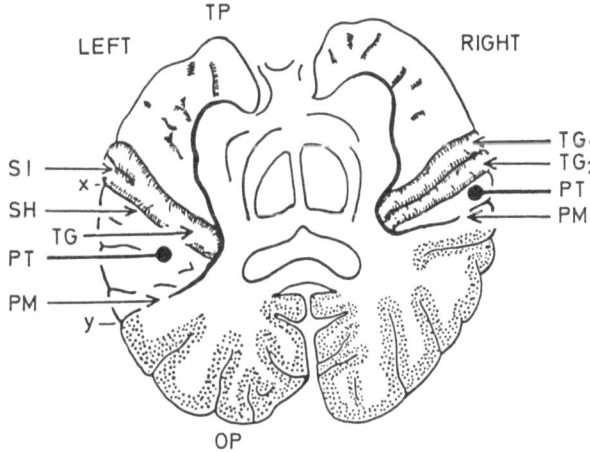

Fig. 1. Upper surfaces of human temporal lobes exposed by a cut on each side in the plane of the Sylvian fissure; anatomical landmarks and typical left-right differences are shown. The posterior margin (*PM*) of the planum temporale (*PT*) slopes backward more sharply on the left than on the right, so that end "y" of the left Sylvian fissure lies posterior to the corresponding point on the right. The anterior margin of the planum formed by the sulcus of Heschl (*SH*) slopes forward more sharply on the left. In this brain there is a single transverse gyrus of Heschl (*TG*) on the left, but two on the right (*TG₁*, *TG₂*). *TP* Temporal pole; *OP* occipital pole; *SI* sulcus intermedius of Beck. Reproduced from Geschwind and Levitsky (1968)

Table 1. *Volume, Cell Density and Cell Numbers of the Temporal Speech Region*

	Right	Left	Differences in %	P
Volume (mm$^3 \times 10^3$)	6.07 ± 0.45	8.40 ± 0.58	38.4	< 0.01
Cell density (n/mm$^3 \times 10^4$)	2.05 ± 0.04	1.99 ± 0.04	2.9	> 0.10
Cell number (n $\times 10^6$)	124.35 ± 9.24	167.42 ± 12.97	34.6	< 0.01

n = 10.

the asymmetry of the brain is genetically inbuilt into the developmental program of the human: by an instruction to generate 40 million more cells on the left side.

Considering the tangential continuity of the neocortex, the definition of the borders of the relevant regions still leave ample freedom for the experimenter to direct the cutting edge of his knife through the depth of the sulci – with a possible difference of several millions more or less nerve cells contained in the excised cortical slabs. There is no way to avoid considerable freedom in subjective judgement. It was imperative, therefore, to design such measurements (more correctly estimates) in double blind experiments, i.e. the workers making the measurements and counts only had code numbers of the excised slabs and the results were evaluated only at the end of the experiments on the basis of the code numbers known only to the experimenter who made the excisions. (In this case to this author; the measurements and calculations were made by Katalin Gallatz under the supervision of Dr. Palkovits. These data are still preliminary and they are published here as a single group of data. Although this study is still far from being finished, however, even these preliminary data are already so interesting, that it is worth while mentioning them. [I do not usually agree to the publication of preliminary results, however, in view of my advanced age and the little likelihood of living to see the data completed, I thought that this exception can be excused.] My sincere thanks are due to Katalin Gallatz and M. Palkovits for graciously letting me use the data at this stage). In making the excisions I took care to make the incisions along the "landmark" sulci in order to "maximize" the cortical slabs on the right side and to "minimize" them on the left. In other words, I was "playing the game" with a consciously introduced bias against the *expected result*.

The results of the measurements and cell counts are shown in Table 1. They are striking, and perhaps even more striking is the exceedingly low standard error, showing that from ten brains used in this study not one significantly deviated from the basic pattern. The

brains were collected randomly from post-mortem procedures performed in the Department of Legal Medicine of Semmelweis University Medical School in adults who suffered (unexpected) sudden death (i.e. without having had specific hospital or medical treatment, probably in the large majority cardiac cases) and in whose history there was no indication of any neurological and/or psychiatric disease. Somebody might ask, of course, whether we did not have any true "right brain speakers" in our sample. But this is unlikely in view of the fact that the vast majority of left-handed people are "left brain speakers" (only about 15–18% of the left-handed being true "right brain speakers") so that the chance of having such an individual in a random sample of ten (10) apparently normal brains is very small.

So there is a clear anatomic substrate for the unique human capacity of the child to begin to acquire the ability of speech in the first (in some individual cases) or on the average in the second year of life.

2. The Biology of Genetically Preprogrammed "Wiring" in Neural Centres

There is ample evidence, mainly in experimental embryology, in favour of the assumption that neuronal connections are genetically preprogrammed. This may go so far as securing very specific functional patterns emerging – by way of "self-organization" – even in total absence of any sensory input. The basic experimental facts were already known much earlier, but, it was only very recently that the true meaning for the entire neural organization began to dawn upon us (Szentágothai: 1984[3]; 1985[4]; 1987a[5]; 1987b[6]; Szentágothai and Érdi, 1989[7]). In view of the experimental facts observed in embryonic transplantation, tissue recombination, and in tissue culturing experiments it is now easily conceivable, that the specific human ability of speech generation and learning is "hard wired" in the Planum temporale, as much as the ability to make stepping movements into the segmental apparatus of the spinal cord.

3. The Neural Mechanism of Speech

The generation of the basic elements of speech – babbling of the infant – are spontaneous and invariable (cross culturally), and so are the deep logical structures of language (Chomsky, 1980[8]).

There is also some evidence (see for example Jesperssen, 1922[9]) that two normal infants left to themselves in a cooperative situation, but otherwise deprived of language spoken in their environment, develop very quickly a personal private language with rather intricate syntactic and grammar rules. Conversely, the so called "wild children" – mainly reared by animals, or otherwise deprived of normal human contact – may acquire a very limited vocabulary later, when returned to normal and helpful human environment, but they become right brain speakers (Curtiss, 1977[10]) and do not ever use speech spontaneously (see also Singh and Zingg, 1939[11]), but only upon command, questioning, and generally only with some coercion. Such wild children have been believed as anecdotal (usually generated by legends), however, the two observations cited remove all possible doubt about their existence. It is important to keep in mind that such "secondary speech" – i.e. learnt in later stages of childhood (say after years 6–10) does not become true human speech, probably because if the "critical functional" developmental period of the left Planum temporale is once missed, the damage is beyond repair. The special experience of the ability to learn American (or Chinese) sign language in deaf-mutes also at later ages, seems to be in good agreement with recent experience with the success of teaching such sign language to anthropoid apes.

The great plasticity of the brain is most impressively demonstrated by the fact that serious damage or loss of the left speech areas at (or shortly after) birth (during fetal development) can be completely compensated (obviously by the right brain).

References

1. Geschwind N, Levitsky W (1968) Science 161: 186–187
2. Witelson SF, Pallie W (1975) Brain 96: 141–146
3. Szentágothai J (1984) Ann Rev Neurosci 7: 1–11
4. Szentágothai J (1985) Naturwissenschaften 72: 303–309
5. Szentágothai J (1987a) In: Blakemore C, Greenfield S (eds) Mindwaves. Blackwell, London, pp 323–326
6. Szentágothai J (1987b) In: Gulyas B (ed) The brain mind problem. Leuven Univ Press, Leuven
7. Szentágothai J, Érdi P (1989) Social Biol Structure 12: 367–384
8. Chomsky N (1980) Rules and Representations. Columbia Univ Press, New York
9. Jesperssen O (1922) Language, its nature, development and origin. London
10. Curtiss S (1977) Genie: A psychologists study of a modern day "Wild Child". Academic Press, New York
11. Singh JAL, Zingg RM (1939) Wolf children and Feral men. Harper Brothers, New York

Correspondence: J. Szentágothai, Institute of Anatomy, Semmelweiss University, Tüzoltó u. 58, H-1450, Budapest, Hungary.

Acta Neurochirurgica (1993) [Suppl] 56: 20–33
© Springer-Verlag 1993

Cortical DC-Potentials in Identification of the Language-Dominant Hemisphere: Linguistical and Clinical Aspects*

E. Altenmüller with collaboration of **W. Kriechbaum, U. Helber, S. Moini, J. Dichgans**, and **D. Petersen**

Department of Neurology, University of Tübingen, Federal Republic of Germany

Summary

In order to find a non-invasive method for determining the hemispheric dominance for language, we studied cortical activation patterns during language processing by means of electrophysiological techniques: DC-potentials were recorded from frontal, central, temporal and parietal electrode positions in 28 right-handed normal subjects and in 16 patients with a history of transient loss of speech and known hemispheric dominance. Subjects were asked to find as many synonyms as possible within 6 seconds to either a concrete or an abstract noun. This task caused a highly significant left-hemispheric lateralization over frontal and central, but not over temporal and parietal cortical areas. Search for synonyms to abstract nouns yielded frontal left-hemispheric dominance in 93% of all normal subjects, search for synonyms to concrete nouns in 85%. Interelectrode correlation coefficients were higher during processing of abstract word categories than during processing of concrete categories. In all patients, frontal and central lateralization corresponded to their hemispheric dominance as determined from clinical data. Advantages as well as inconveniences of this technique are discussed and compared to other invasive and noninvasive tools of assessing speech lateralization.

Keywords: Hemispheric dominance; cortical DC-Potentials; language processing; semantic categories.

Introduction

Can the WADA-test be replaced by non-invasive methods? Up to now, the intracarotid sodium amytal procedure[27,28] is the most commonly used diagnostic tool for determining speech dominance prior to neurosurgical treatment. The necessity for exact knowledge of a patient's language-dominance arose after the introduction of neurosurgical treatment of chronic drug resistant seizures comprising e.g. unilateral removal of the temporal lobe[11]. Since this kind of operation has to be modified when the language dominant hemisphere is involved[10], preoperative assessment of dominance is crucial. However, the Wadatest used for this purpose has some disadvantages: the method is invasive, carries some degree of physical risk and is uncomfortable to the patients. Sometimes the procedure is difficult to administer and the results remain unclear[17]. Finally, since normative data usually are obtained in patients with epilepsy one has to be cautious about generalizing from the data to healthy subjects.

In the past decade, two alternative methods of dominance-determination have been introduced into clinical practice: the measurement of regional cerebral blood flow[20] and the measurement of cerebral metabolism[14]. Since both methods rely on the administration of radioactive tracer substances they are – like the WADA-test – invasive and their applicability is limited in patients as well as in healthy subjects. Furthermore, the required expensive equipment is not available at all medical centers.

Searching for non-invasive means of assessing speech lateralization, we started to study the distribution of the cortical DC-potential shifts related to language processing[16]. The rationale behind this approach was, that cortical activation lasting for more than 2 s is accompanied by an increase of surface negativity[8] caused by sustained postsynaptic depolarisation of larger populations of cortical neurons. Measuring the resulting local changes of cortical DC-potential should therefore provide a tool for the cerebral localization of higher mental functions. Because significant changes in DC-potentials develop comparatively slowly, the design of cognitive paradigms has to ensure a steady cognitive activity of at least two seconds duration. The resulting cortical activation causes DC-potentials of high amplitudes (30 μV) over those areas engaged in the specific

---
* Supported by a grant from the Deutsche Forschungsgesellschaft (SFB 307)

task which topographically correlate to the "classical" localization sites as determined from lesion studies. In a series of studies we investigated the language dominance in right-handed and left-handed healthy subjects confirming the left-hemispheric speech-dominance in the large majority of both, right-handers and left-handers[1,2,3].

The purpose of the present study was twofold. Firstly, we attempted to improve our method of speech-dominance assessment by varying the paradigms: from dichotic listening studies[9] it is argued, that left-hemispheric lateralization is more pronounced during processing of words with abstract semantic content than in processing of concrete, highly imageable words. Detailed neuropsychological studies provide evidence for selective impairment or preservation of different semantic categories in aphasics[13] and in patients suffering from global amnesic syndromes due to herpes simplex encephalitis[29]. These studies, indicating a categorial specificity in lexical processing, encouraged us to compare cerebral activation patterns during processing of concrete and abstract semantic material.

The second aim was an external validation of our method. Since we were not able to apply the WADA-test as a reference method in our subjects we studied a group of patients with known hemispheric speech-dominance from clinical data. These patients presented with a history of transient loss or severe impairment of speech due to well defined unilateral cortical dysfunction occurring in most cases during the course of transient ischemic attacks or classic migraine.

Methods

Healthy Subjects, Patients, Tasks and Recording Procedure

Twenty-eight male right-handed healthy subjects between 21 and 51 years of age (mean 28.7) and sixteen patients aged from 15 to 67 years (mean 43.5) with a history of transient impairment of speech were investigated. All healthy subjects as well as fourteen patients scored 100% dextrality according to the Edinburgh handedness inventory[18]. Two patients were left-handers.

In all patients, the clinical symptoms referring to speech impairment did not last longer than 3 days. All recordings were performed, when the patients had no more detectable language deficits and were in a good general condition. The clinical data are summarized in Table 1.

The language task demanded in subjects and patients was the search for synonyms to a spoken noun either with concrete or with abstract semantical content. All stimuli were common objects or abstract expressions (see Appendix). Abstract and concrete nouns were presented in a random sequence.

Each trial started with an acoustic signal that prompted the subject to fixate a point in order to avoid artifacts caused by eye-movements. After the fixation movement, the measurement was started and a baseline was established by recording 3 s of cortical activity without stimulation (preperiod). A tone-signal indicated the beginning of the stimulus-period of 2 s duration during which a word was spoken to the subject. This stimulus-period was followed by a 4 s task-period during which the subjects had to search "mentally" for as many synonyms as possible. A final tone signal indicated the end of the task-period. Since tongue movements lead to artifacts, oral communication of the synonyms found was not allowed until the end of each measurement. Including time for electrode-positioning, an experimental session took around 2 hours.

To obtain data on the intra-individual reproducibility of task-related patterns of potential-shifts, we repeated the recording procedure in 10 normal subjects in the same experimental session.

Data Acquisition

DC-Potentials were recorded from the scalp by nonpolarizable AgCl-electrodes (impedance below 3 kOhms), positioned according to the Jasper 10/20 system over F_3/F_4, C_3/C_4, T_3/T_4 and P_3/P_4. Unipolar leads with linked earlobes as a reference as well as horizontal electro-oculogram (HEOG), vertical electro-oculogram (VEOG) and galvanic skin response (GSR) were recorded.

The signals were amplified using DC-amplifiers with externally triggered DC-compensation (Tönnies, Freiburg, upper cut off 10 Hz). For artifact control, all traces were monitored on a 16 channel ink-writer (Nihon–Kohden 4317-FG). Only trials without eye-movements, sweating artifacts, and larger DC-drifts ($>100\,\mu V/min$) during which the subject found at least one synonymous or closely related noun were accepted for averaging. Data were sampled and stored using a micro-processor board (INTEL iSPC 386-16 with DT 2801 A). From each subject or patient, 30–60 trials were averaged.

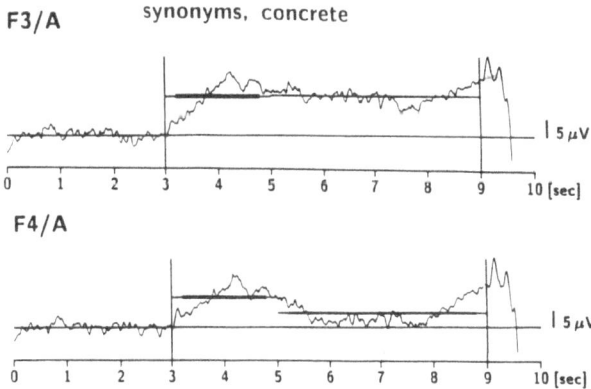

Fig. 1. Averaged traces (20 trials) of left (F_3) and right frontal leads (F_4) for a normal subject during search for synonyms. The data are displayed according to the conventions used for EEG-recordings (negativity pointing upwards). After the pre-period (0–3 s), during which only fixation is required, an acoustic signal indicates the beginning of the 2-s stimulus-period (first vertical bar) during which the words are presented acoustically. The subsequent 4-s task-period is terminated by a second acoustic signal (second vertical bar). Surface negativity increases in both electrodes during the stimulus-period but the activation persists during the task period almost only over the left hemisphere, indicating a left-hemispheric dominance for the required task. Horizontal bars show mean amplitude during the periods +/− standard error

Table 1. *Clinical Data, Diagnosis, Character and Duration of Symptoms in Patients with Transient Loss of Speech*

Case	Sex	Age	Diagnosis	Character of symptoms and results of additional examinations	Duration of symptoms
Right-handed patients					
F.K.	f	17.3	c.m.	motor aphasia, right-sided hemiparesis, hemihypaesthesia, left-frontal headache, EEG normal.	14 hs
K.D.	f	18.6	c.m.	motor aphasia, right-sided hemiparesis, left-frontal headache, 3–4 Hz focus in the EEG.	10 hs
T.L.	m	15.1	c.m.	amnesic aphasia, right-sided hemihypaesthesia, left-sided headache, left temporal 3–5 Hz EEG-focus.	4 hs
M.S.	m	17.2	c.m.	global aphasia, right-sided hemiparesis, left fronto-temporal headache, left frontal 6–7 Hz EEG-focus.	5 hs
I.H.	f	60.2	tia	motor aphasia, right-sided hemiparesis, 90% stenosis of the left internal carotid artery. EEG and CT-scan normal.	1 h
H.B.	f	65.8	tia	motor aphasia, right-sided hemiparesis. 90% stenosis of the left internal carotid artery. EEG and CT normal.	18 hs
G.L.	m	64.7	tia	sensory aphasia, right-sided hemiparesis. 50% stenosis of the left internal carotid artery. EEG and CT normal.	15 min
G.K.	m.	64.8	tia	motor aphasia, right-sided hemiparesis. 90% stenosis of the left internal carotid artery. EEG and CT normal.	15 min
I.H.	f	50.5	P.R.I.N.D.	global aphasia, right-sided hemiparesis and hypaesthesia. Doppler-sonography and EEG normal, CT-scan: small left temporo-polar hypo-density of 3 cm in diameter.	48 hs
W.S.	m	40.3	P.R.I.N.D.	motor aphasia, right-sided hemiparesis. Doppler-sonography, EEG, CT and angiography normal. Persistent latent hemi-paresis on the right side during six months.	56 hs
M.K.	m	53.9	P.R.I.N.D.	motor aphasia, right-sided hemiparesis. Doppler-sonography, EEG and CT-scan normal.	48 hs
K.K.	m	46.6	P.R.I.N.D.	sensory aphasia, right-sided hemihypaesthesia. Doppler-sonography and EEG normal. CT-scan: left temporo-parietal hypo-density. Cardiac arrhythmia.	48 hs
A.K.	m	67.2	P.R.I.N.D.	sensory aphasia, no motor signs. Doppler-sonography normal. Left temporo-parietal 5–7 Hz EEG-focus. CT scan: left parieto-occipital hypodensity of 3 cm in diameter.	72 hs
R.R.	m	26.6	traumatic bleeding	sensory aphasia, dyscalculia, no motor signs. Left parietal 5–7 Hz focus. CT-scan: intracerebral parietal bleeding of 3 cm in diameter.	48 hs
Left-handed patients					
B.S.	f	29.3	angioma	attacks of amnesic aphasia in 1980 and 1989. No neurological deficits on admission. Left temporal angioma. Postoperatively amnesic aphasia.	5–10 min
H.W.	m	45.2	angioma	Grand-mal seizures. Aura with amnesic aphasia. No neurological deficits on admission. Right temporal angioma.	5–15 min

c.m. = classic migraine, tia = transient ischaemic attack, P.R.I.N.D. = prolonged reversible ischaemic deficit.

Figure 1 shows averaged data for one subject from the two frontal leads (F_3, F_4) exemplifying the periods used for further data-analysis.

Methodological Limitations in Patients

In 10 patients, only 8 DC-amplifiers were available. Since vertical and horizontal eye movements had to be recorded simultaneously, we were limited to 6 DC-recordings over both hemispheres. In these cases the electrode positions used were according to the Jasper 10/20 system F_3/F_4, C_3/C_4 and PT_3/PT_4 (midway between P_3/P_4 and T_3/T_4).

To keep the recording procedure as short as possible, only search for synonyms to concrete word categories was investigated. In two patients, we were forced to exclude frontal electrodes from averaging because of artifacts due to sweating (Patients GK and GL).

Further Data Processing and Statistical Analysis

All data were normalized by equating the mean of the preperiod with zero. Small linear DC-drifts ($< 100 \mu V/min$) which often occur during DC-recordings were estimated from a linear regression over the preperiod and subtracted from the data.

To describe the event-related slow potential shifts, mean values during stimulus- and task-period were calculated and compared with the preperiod by analysis of variance. Lateralization was assessed by comparing the corresponding electrode-positions over the left and right hemisphere, using a paired ANOVA. To derive group-statistics the data on activation as well as those on lateralization were dichotomized (positive shift vs. negative shift in mean value; left-hemispheric mean vs. right-hemispheric mean) and tested as Bernoulli trials for departure from equal probability (two-sided test). Group inter-electrode correlation coefficients were calculated for the mean values during stimulus-period and task-period as a measure of co-activation of different cortical areas.

Results in Normal Subjects

Figure 2 shows the grand averages over all subjects during search for synonyms to concrete (dotted lines) and abstract nouns (solid lines). In all electrode-positions, the potential-shifts begin with a large bilateral negativation during the 2 s stimulus-period, followed during the task-period by a sustained plateau-like potential over the left frontal, central and temporal leads. For the grand-averages, the statistically significant differences between the two stimulus-conditions can be summarized as follows: In the right frontal and right temporal leads (F_4, T_4) search for synonyms to concrete semantic categories cause a larger activation than abstract semantic categories do. On the other hand, in

the left parietal lead (P_3) abstract nouns yield a larger negativation than concrete nouns do.

The inter-individual variations of mean potential shifts can better be estimated from scatter-plots shown in Fig. 3. For the stimulus condition "abstract", the mean DC-potential amplitudes during the task-period over the left frontal vs. right frontal and over the left temporal vs. right temporal electrode locations are displayed. These plots allow one to assess the activation (negativation or positivation) of both electrodes as well as cortical lateralization in individual subjects (cf. Fig. 3 leg.).

Table 2 summarizes the mean amplitudes of DC-potential shifts (µV) and the standard-deviation (sd) for both, stimulus- (S) and task-period (T) during the search for synonyms to concrete and abstract nouns. The mean amplitudes of DC-potential shifts do not differ significantly in the different stimulus conditions (pairwise t-test, $\alpha = .01$). Standard deviations are in all

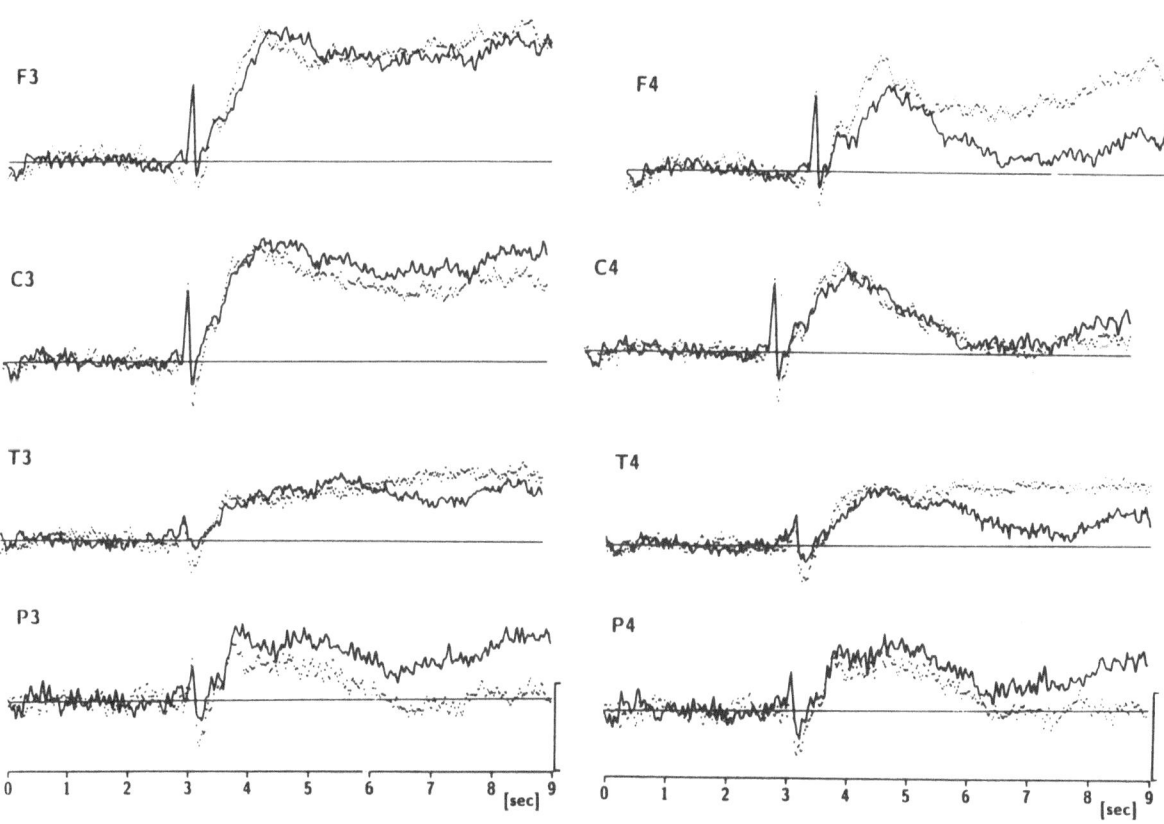

Fig. 2. Grand-averages over all 28 normal subjects during search for synonyms to abstract nouns (solid lines) and to concrete nouns (dotted lines). Recordings from electrodes over the left frontal (F_3), central (C_3), temporal (T_3) and parietal (P_3) brain areas are displayed on the left side, recordings over the right hemisphere on the right side. Calibration bars plotted on the right side of the time-base correspond to 10 µVs. The acoustical signal indicating the beginning of the stimulus period yields an evoked potential (N 100) visible in all recordings. Subsequently, surface negativity increases bilaterally. During the task-period, highest amplitudes of DC-potential persist over left-frontal (F_3) and -central (C_3) brain areas. Comparing both stimulus conditions, concrete nouns yield a higher activation over right frontal (F_4) and right temporal (T_4) brain areas whereas abstract nouns cause higher activation over left parietal (P_3) brain regions

synonyms, abstract

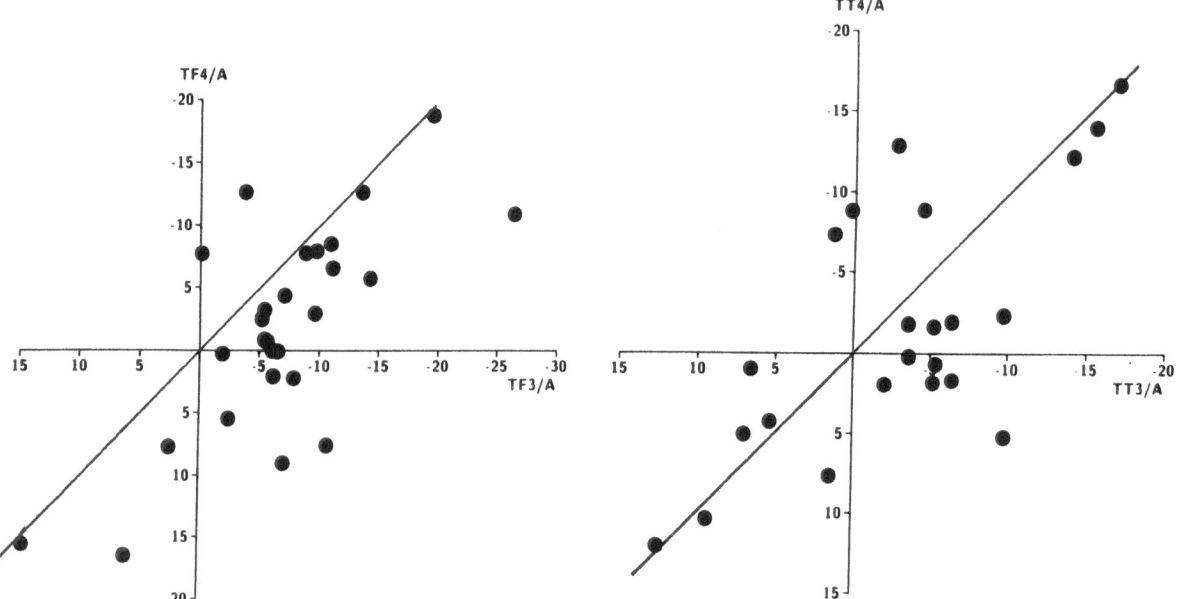

Fig. 3. Scatter-plots of mean amplitudes (μV) of DC-potential during the task period of stimulus condition "abstract": On the left values of left frontal (x-axis, F_3) vs. right frontal (y-axis, F_4) activity are displayed. On the right, values of left temporal (x-axis T_3) vs. right temporal (T_4) are shown. Each dot represents one subject. Left-hemispheric lateralization is plotted below, right-hemispheric lateralization above the diagonal. Note the large interindividual variation of values ranging from $-25\,\mu Vs$ to $+15\,\mu Vs$

electrode positions larger during the task period than during the stimulus period.

Polarity of DC-Shifts

The data on polarity of DC-shifts during stimulus (ST) and task period (T) are shown in Fig. 4 and summarized in Table 3. There is no significant difference in polarity between the two stimulus-conditions. Both stimulus-conditions yield the same basic patterns: generally the probability of negativation is higher during the stimulus period than during the task period. During the task period, the probability of negativation is higher over the left than over the right hemisphere with the only exception of the right parietal electrode (P_4). Furthermore probability of negativation is higher during abstract than during concrete synonym searching.

In the 10 healthy subjects recorded repeatedly in one experimental session, the pattern of polarity remained identical in both recordings for both stimulus conditions.

Lateralization

As with polarity the two stimulus conditions yield basically the same results (Fig. 5): there is a significant left-hemispheric lateralization effect in frontal and

central electrode positions but not in temporal and parietal locations. This holds for both, stimulus-period as well as task-period. The data are summarized in Table 4: Left-hemispheric lateralization is more probable during search for abstract than during search for concrete synonyms. The highest percentage of lateralization to the left hemisphere occurred over frontal regions with 93% for the condition "abstract nouns" and 85% for condition "concrete nouns".

In the 10 healthy subjects recorded repeatedly, the data on lateralization were qualitatively reproduced in all electrode positions. The quantitative "degree" of lateralization however, as determined in μVs (left- vs. right-hemisphere negativation or positivation) varied inbetween both measurements.

Inter-Electrode Correlation

A marked difference related to the two stimulus conditions was revealed by calculation of second-order properties of the data. Whereas in the stimulus condition "concrete" each electrode site was significantly ($\alpha = 0.1$) correlated with 3.25 electrode positions in the average, interelectrode correlation was markedly higher in the stimulus condition "abstract". During this condition, each electrode site was correlated with 6.25 electrode positions in the average (Fig. 6).

Table 2. *Mean Amplitudes* (µVs) *of DC-Potential-Shift in Relation to the Preperiod* (*Mean*) *and Standard Deviation* (sd) *calculated for each Electrode during Stimulus-* (S) *and Task-Period* (T) *and for each Stimulus Condition*

Age	Normal subjects 21–51 ($\varnothing = 28.5$ years) Synonyms concrete		Synonyms abstract			Right-handed patients 15–67 ($\varnothing = 43.5$ years) Synonyms concrete	
	mean	sd	mean	sd		mean	sd
F3 S	−4.6	2.5	−4.7	3.3		−7.8	4.0
F3 T	−6.7	4.8	−6.5	8.1		−14.2	9.0
F4 S	−3.0	3.5	−2.9	3.2		−4.2	3.0
F4 T	−2.5	6.2	−1.5	8.2		−6.0	7.4
C3 S	−4.1	2.8	−4.4	2.4		−6.7	2.7
C3 T	−4.4	5.6	+5.5	6.5		−10.2	7.9
C4 S	−2.7	2.8	−2.9	3.0		−5.0	4.7
C4 T	−1.0	5.8	−1.9	8.1		−4.7	6.8
T3 S	−1.5	1.9	−1.8	2.8	*PT3 S	−3.5	1.5
T3 T	−3.4	5.2	−3.6	6.7	PT3 T	−4.1	5.9
T4 S	−1.5	3.5	−1.3	2.7	PT4 S	−2.8	3.0
T4 T	−2.3	6.1	−2.8	7.9	PT4 T	−3.4	5.6
P3 S	−1.3	2.6	−2.3	2.8			
P3 T	−0.3	6.0	−2.7	6.6			
P4 S	−1.5	3.1	−2.3	3.4			
P4 T	−0.5	6.2	−2.8	7.5			

* In 10 patients, for technical reasons parieto-temporal recordings were performed.

Table 3. *Data on Polarity in Normal Subjects and in Right-Handed Patients*

Stimulus	F3		F4		C3		C4		T3		T4		P3		P4	
	−	+	−	+	−	+	−	+	−	+	−	+	−	+	−	+
Concrete	26	1	25	2	27	1	23	5	21	3	17	6	17	7	16	8
Abstract	27	1	23	5	28	0	24	4	17	7	18	6	21	3	20	4
									PT3		PT4					
									−	+	−	+				
Patients	12	0	11	1	14	0	12	2	10	0	9	1				

Task	F3		F4		C3		C4		T3		T4		P3		P4	
	−	+	−	+	−	+	−	+	−	+	−	+	−	+	−	+
Concrete	25	2	18	9	23	5	18	10	18	6	16	7	11	13	13	11
Abstract	24	4	16	12	23	5	15	13	17	7	13	11	17	7	17	7
									PT3		PT4					
									−	+	−	+				
Patients	12	0	10	2	12	2	11	3	7	3	8	2				

Absolute values (number of ss or patients) are indicated. Missing values are due to data which had to be excluded from further data-processing because of artifacts.

Recordings in Patients

Clinical Data (Summarized in Table 1)

All right-handed patients had left-hemispheric speech-dominance according to clinical data: Four patients had attacks of classic migraine with aphasia, right-sided hemihypaesthesia and/or hemiparesis and left-sided headache.

Nine patients suffered from transient ischaemic attacks or prolonged reversible ischaemic neurological deficits (P.R.I.N.D.) due to cerebrovascular diseases. During their attacks, aphasia was accompanied by right-sided hemiparesis or hemihypaesthesia. Three of these patients (I.H., K.K., A.K.) were asymptomatic when investigated in our study, but revealed hypodensities in the left temporo-parietal area in CT-scan due to small infarctions. DC-traces of patient A.K. are shown in Fig. 7.

Patient R.R. presented during two days with symptoms of sensory aphasia and dyscalculia caused by a closed head injury accompanied by a left parietal traumatic haematoma 3 cm in diameter.

The two left-handed patients (B.S., H.E.) suffered from intracranial arterio-venous angiomas. Patient B.S., on admission to our hospital in 1989 aged 29 years, first exhibited symptoms in 1980 when she was presented with a short attack of vertigo and amnesic aphasia of several minutes followed by a loss of consciousness lasting about

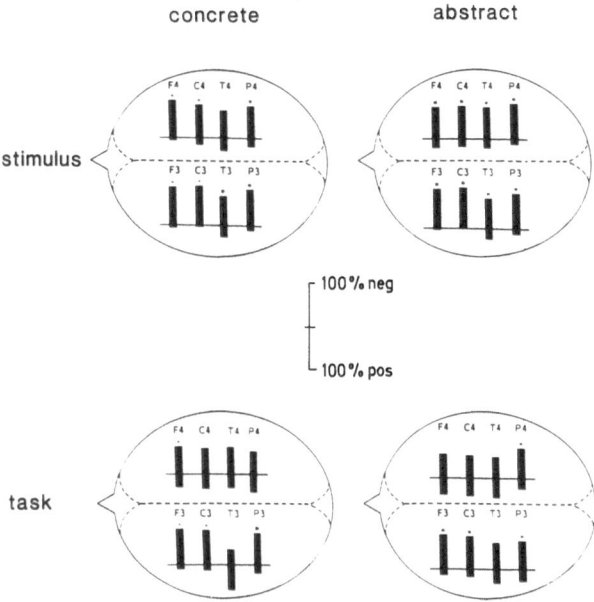

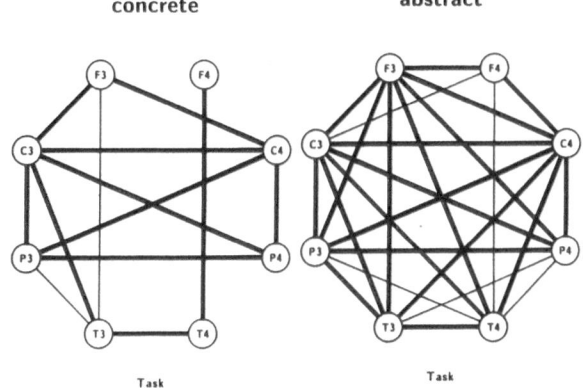

Fig. 6. Inter-electrode correlation diagram for the task period during stimulus condition "*concrete*" (left side) and stimulus condition "*abstract*" (right side). Thick bars show a significant correlation at $\alpha = 0.01$, thin bars at $\alpha = 0.05$

Fig. 4. Dichotomic representation of group statistics referring to polarity during stimulus condition "*concrete*" (left side) and stimulus condition "*abstract*" (right side) for each electrode-position. Negativation points upwards, positivation points downwards. Statistics are calculated for the stimulus-period (upper half) and the task-period (lower half). Significant departures from chance level are marked with an asteriks ("*"$\alpha = 0.01$)

Table 4. *Data on Lateralization in Normal Subjects and in Right-Handed Patients.* Absolute Values are Indicated

Stimulus	Frontal		Central		Temporal		Parietal	
	left	right	left	right	left	right	left	right
Concrete	23	4	20	8	13	10	12	12
Abstract	23	6	22	6	14	10	13	11
					Parietotemporal			
					left	right +		
Patients	12	0	13	1	7	3		

Task	Frontal		Central		Temporal		Parietal	
	left	right	left	right	left	right	left	right
Concrete	23	4	24	4	14	9	10	10
Abstract	26	2	23	5	15	9	11	13
					Parietotemporal			
					left	right +		
Patients	12	0	14	0	6	4		

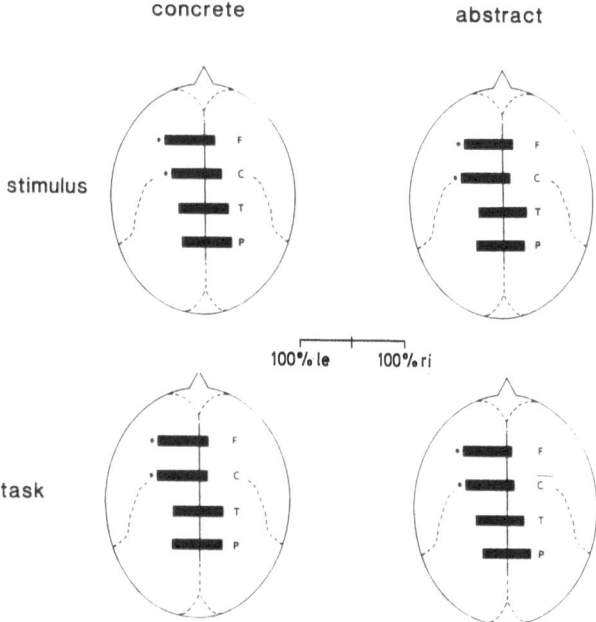

Fig. 5. Dichotomic representation of group statistics referring to lateralization during stimulus condition "*concrete*" (left side) and stimulus condition "*abstract*". Left-hemispheric lateralization points to the left side, right-hemispheric lateralization to the right side. Statistics are calculated for the stimulus-period (upper half) and the task-period (lower half). Significant deviations from chance level are marked with an asteriks ("*", $\alpha = 0.01$)

4 hours. A similar attack had occurred in 1984. On admission neurological and neuropsychological examination was normal. The handedness inventory revealed 60% sinistrality. She reported, that she wrote and painted primarily with the left hand as a preschool child, but was trained to use the right hand during the first years of primary school. MR-scan (Fig. 8) and angiography revealed an arterio-venous malformation of about 4 cm in diameter located in the left temporo-parietal lobe. DC-potentials were recorded before the operation. (Fig. 9). After operation, she developed amnesic aphasia caused by a secondary bleeding into the operation site. Fortunately, she recovered completely from aphasia during a one year follow-up.

Patient HW, aged 45 years was admitted to our department in 1989 with a history of six generalized tonic-clonic epileptic seizures during the past 11 years. The seizures were regularly preceded by an aura with amnesic aphasia during a period of several minutes. On admission, neurological and neuropsychological examination was normal. Handedness index yielded 100% sinistrality. Routine EEG showed a 3–4 Hz focus over the right temporo-parietal region. MR-scan (Fig. 10) and angiography revealed a large *right* temporal

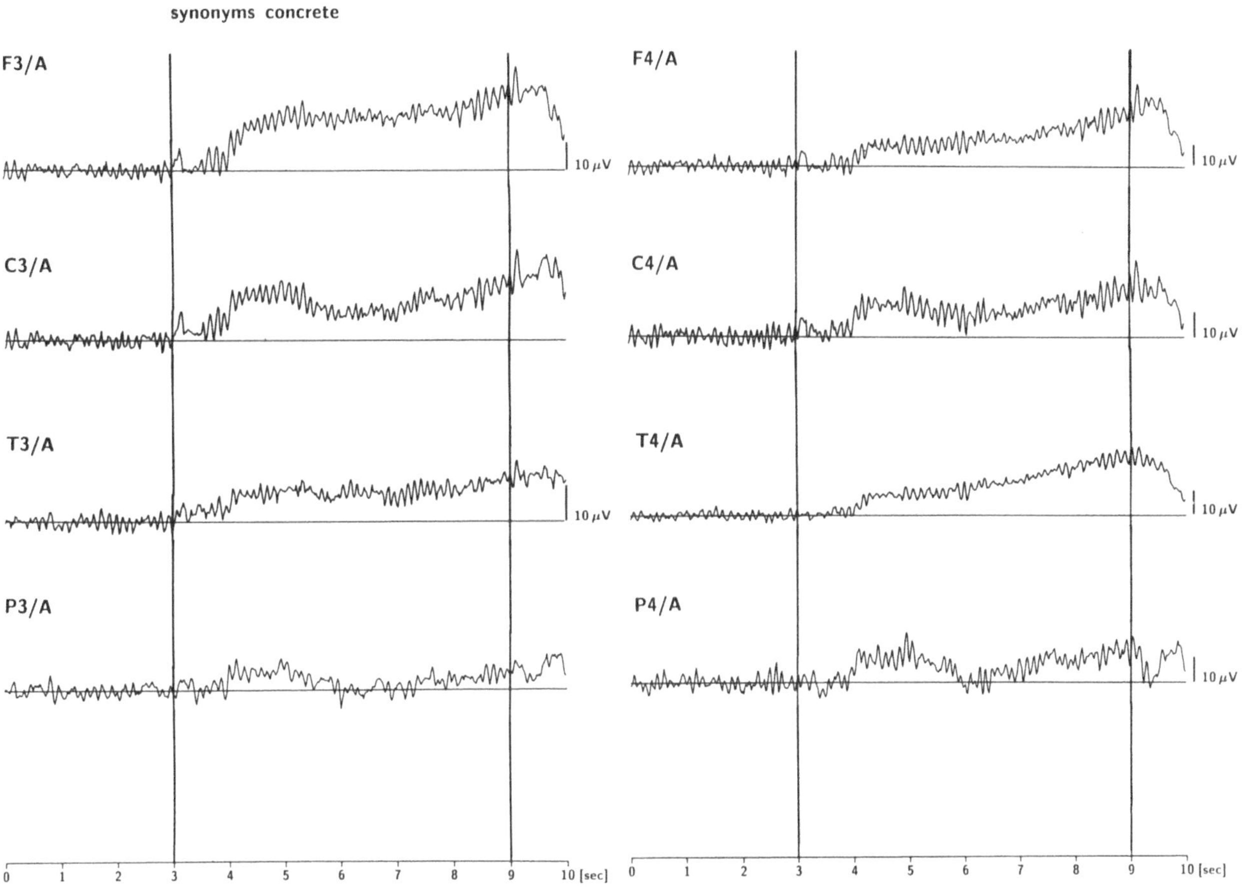

synonyms concrete

F3/A

C3/A

T3/A

P3/A

F4/A

C4/A

T4/A

P4/A

10 μV

10 μV

10 μV

10 μV

10 μV

10 μV

10 μV

10 μV

0 1 2 3 4 5 6 7 8 9 10 [sec]

0 1 2 3 4 5 6 7 8 9 10 [sec]

Fig. 7. DC-recordings of patient AK: 25 trials during stimulus condition "synonyms concrete" are averaged. Same nomenclature as in Fig. 2. Bilateral activation occurs in frontal, central and temporal recordings, preponderance of negativity over the left hemisphere occurs in frontal and central leads, indicating a left-hemispheric dominance for language functions

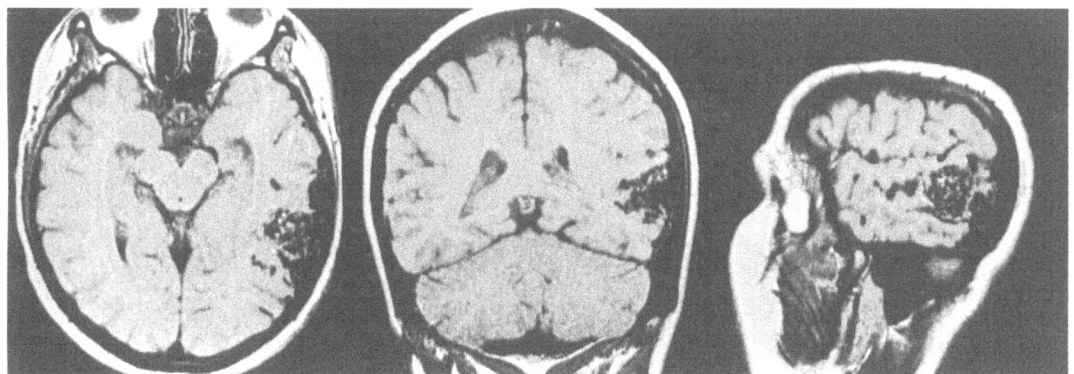

Fig. 8. T_1-weighted MR-images of patient BS (1.5 T, TR = 600 ms, TE = 15 ms) revealing a left temporal arteriovenous angioma

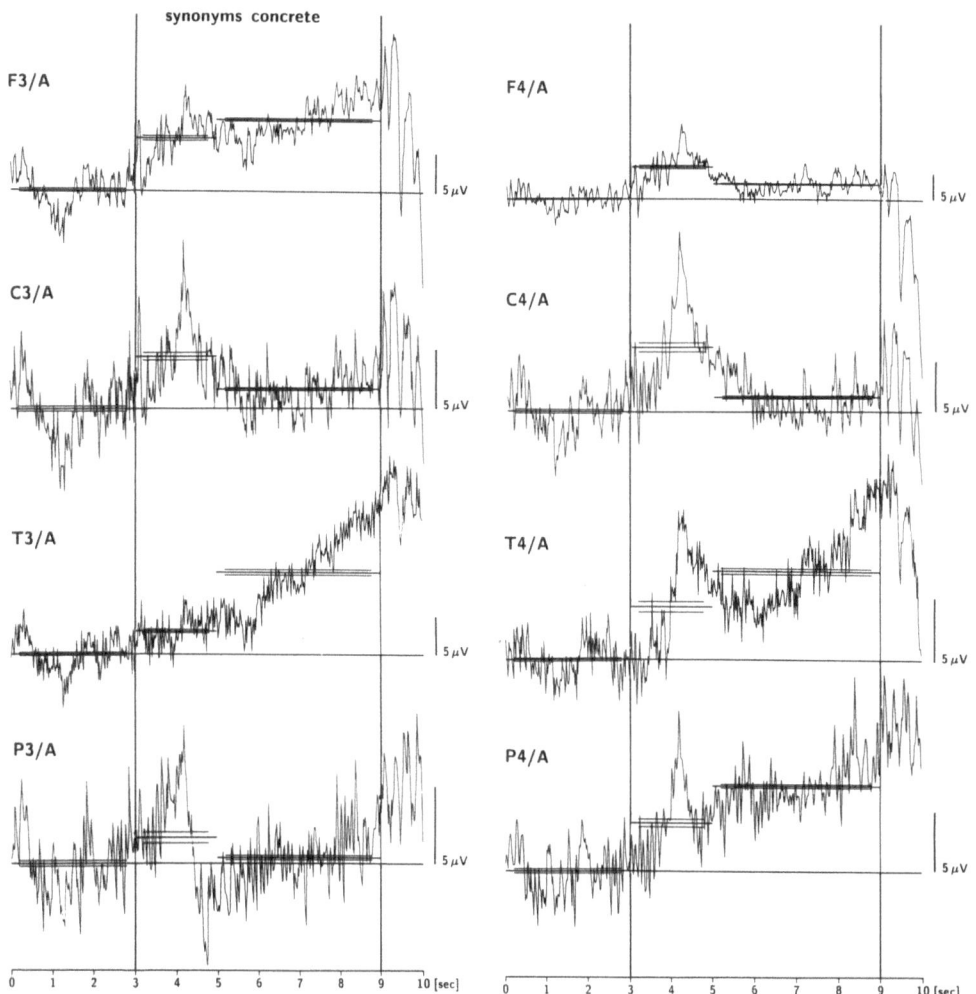

Fig. 9. DC-recordings of patient BS: Superposition of high frequencies as "noise" due to the small number of averaged trials (n = 12). In frontal leads, clear left-hemispheric dominance results. Note atypical trace in the left-temporal recording (T_3) with missing negativation during the stimulus period as a possible correlate to the structural lesion in the underlying brain area

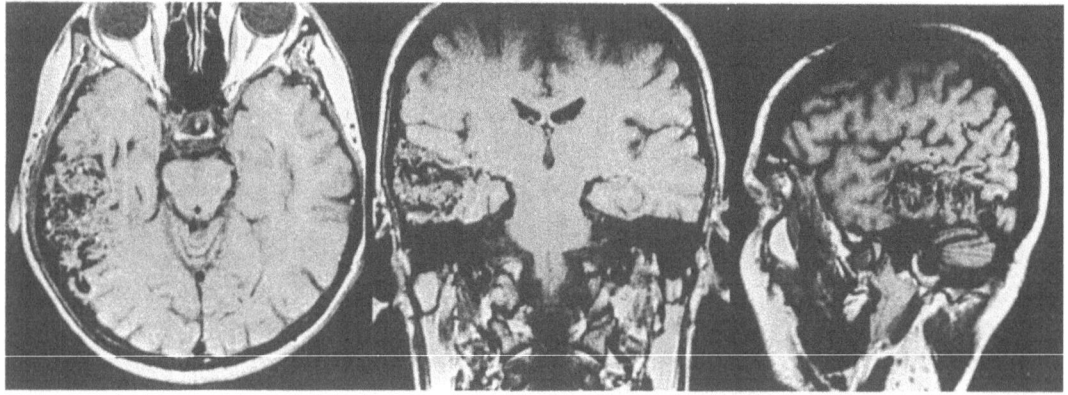

Fig. 10. T_1-weighted MR-images of patient HW (1.5 T, TR = 600 ms, TE = 15 ms) revealing a right temporal arteriovenous angioma

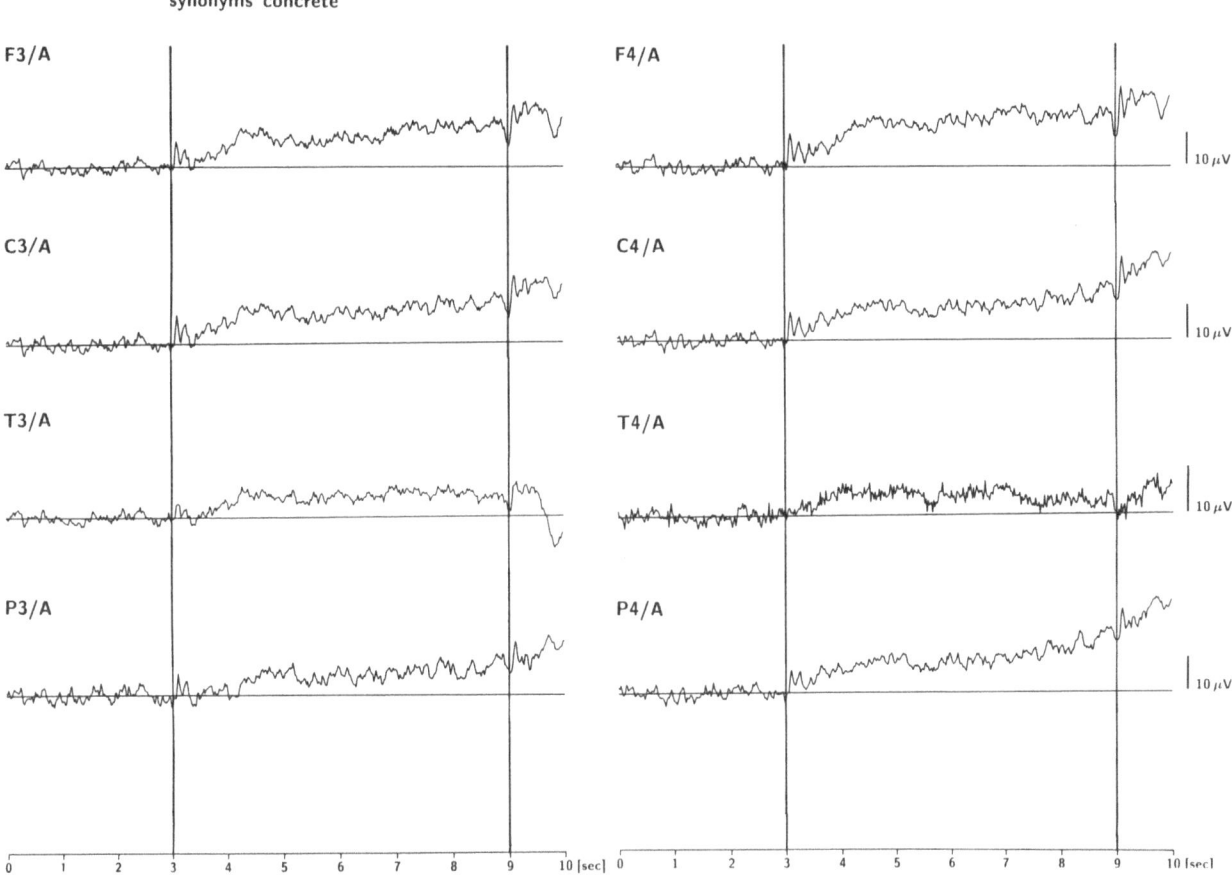

Fig. 11. DC-traces of patient HW revealing preponderance of activation over the right frontal (F_4) brain areas, indicating a right-hemispheric dominance for language in this left-handed patient

arterio-venous malformation of 5×6 cm in diameter. In this patient, according to clinical evidence, right-hemispheric speech-dominance must be assumed.

Results in Patients

In frontal and central leads, all right-handed patients showed left-hemispheric lateralization but in parieto-temporal leads, lateralization to the left and to the right hemisphere was equally probable. That means, that only the lateralization in frontal and central leads is correlated to the language-dominant hemisphere as determined from clinical data. Concerning the polarity of DC-potential-shifts, most patients yielded an increase of negativity in frontal and central leads, as observed in normal subjects.

As a representative example, Fig. 7 shows the recording of patient A.K., presenting a clear left-hemispheric lateralization of surface negativity during both, stimulus and task-period in frontal and central leads. Mean values and standard-deviations for the 14 right-handed patients are listed in Table 2 (right column), data on polarity are summarized in Table 3.

Data referring to lateralization are listed in Table 4. In frontal and central leads all right-handed patients revealed left-hemispheric lateralization during the task-period.

The recordings of the two left-handed patients are shown in Figs. 9 and 11: Patient BS (Fig. 9) exhibits a clear preponderance of surface negativity over the left fronto-central region, confirming her left-hemispheric speech dominance. In contrast, the DC-recording of patient HW (Fig. 11) revealed a right-hemispheric preponderance of negativation over frontal and central leads as expected from clinical data. This patient is one of the rare examples of right-hemispheric speech in a left-hander.

Discussion

The present study was designed to improve and to validate our method of identifying the language-dominant hemisphere. The main results may be summarized as follows:

1) DC-potentials during language-processing reveal

significant left-hemispheric lateralization only in frontal and central, but not in temporal and parietal brain areas. The fronto-central lateralization in patients with transient impairment of speech is concordant with the "true" hemispheric-dominance as determined from clinical data.

2) The stimulus conditions "abstract" and "concrete" do not differ significantly with respect to lateralization and polarity when tested as subject-based Bernoulli-trials. The grand-averages reveal a pronounced right-frontal and -temporal activation during search for synonyms to concrete nouns and a left-parietal activation during search for abstract nouns. A further difference between the two stimulus conditions is the higher inter-electrode correlation during processing of abstract semantic categories.

3) Language processing does not exclusively cause sustained negativation of cortical DC-potentials: Positivation, especially over right-hemispheric parietal and temporal areas occurs frequently.

4) Cortical activation patterns during language processing are not uniform but vary from individual to individual. Intra-individually however, the activation patterns remain stable.

*Lateralization of DC-shifts: Evidence
of Left-Hemispheric Language-Dominance
in Right-Handers*

The most constant finding common to normal subjects and to patients is the fronto-central lateralization with activation of BROCA's area. This can be explained by our paradigm: "mental" search for synonyms is accompanied by "silent" speech, i.e. the subject is silently formulating the synonyms found. This cognitive operation is not subject to any cognitive "strategy" since it represents the final common path of speech production, regardless if a word is said aloud or silently. As is known from cerebral blood-flow studies, silent speech is accompanied by a maximal activation of left fronto-central language area[15]. From the 100% concordance of fronto-central lateralization with "true" speech-dominance as determined from clinical evaluations in patients with transient loss of speech, we conclude that cortical DC-potentials reliably reflect hemispheric dominance for language, provided that appropriate paradigms and stimuli are applied.

Surprisingly, the WERNICKE-area (left-temporal and parieto-temporal electrode positions), which was expected to contribute to the decoding of the semantic material and to the lexical processing was not

significantly activated during both, stimulus- and task-period. In an attempt to explain the absence of left-temporal dominance, one could argue, that activation of the WERNICKE-area, especially the planum temporale could be missed by our recording procedure: since the electrical dipoles are positioned rectangularly to the cortical surface, activation of the planum temporale projects electrically to central leads, i.e. C_z and P_z. Moreover, it may play a role that immediately after or even during the perception of a presented stimulus subsequent cognitive processes such as short-time storage of the stimulus, visual associations, access to the verbal memory etc. begin; these cognitive operations certainly influence lateralization over temporal and parietal areas.

*Semantic Content of Stimuli and Cortical
Activation Patterns*

Cortical activation patterns during both stimulus conditions did not differ significantly with respect to polarity and lateralization when tested on a single-subject basis. This lack of significancies is due to the large interindividual variability of activation patterns most probably caused by individually different strategies when solving the required tasks. It should be emphasized that, as far as investigations of hemispheric dominance in individual persons are concerned, the stimulus-condition may play an important role: Two of the 28 normal subjects exhibited right hemispheric dominance during the stimulus condition "concrete" and left hemispheric dominance during the condition "abstract". From dichotic listening studies, it has been argued that words with concrete semantic content might be processed to a higher degree in the right hemisphere compared to words with abstract semantic content[9]. The more pronounced right-frontal and right-temporal activation during search for synonyms to concrete nouns in the present study supports this hypothesis of a category specific processing of verbal material in both hemispheres.

At present, assessment of speech-dominance remains uncertain in subjects with different lateralization during different language-tasks. However, the incidence of left-hemispheric dominance during search for synonyms to abstract nouns corresponds with 93% closely to results obtained from lesion-studies (95–99% according to[19]) and from WADA-tests (94% according to[17]), much closer than the 85% obtained in the stimulus condition "concrete".

A clear stimulus-related group-effect was a striking change in *correlation pattern* with enormous increase of inter-electrode correlation during search for synonyms to abstract nouns when compared to concrete nouns. Generally, inter-electrode correlation can be considered as an indicator of inter- and intra-hemispheric connectivity[12,25]. Since in the present study correlation was only calculated as a group-effect within all 28 normal subjects but not within the data obtained in single individuals, conclusions should be drawn cautiously. We interpret the higher inter-electrode correlation during search for abstract nouns as an unspecific effect most probably related to task-difficulty: A high degree of task-difficulty causes synchronous activation of large cortical areas comprising both hemispheres[6,21]. Such high-grade synchronized activation or inhibition of large cortical areas leads to an increase of inter-electrode correlation as observed in the present paradigm. This interpretation is supported by the fact that most subjects found it more difficult to search synonyms to abstract nouns than to concrete nouns when asked informally.

*Activation or Inhibition: Polarity
of DC-Potentials*

Cortical activation leads to negativation, cortical inhibition to positivation of DC-potentials – at least when recorded from the surface of the cortex[8]. Epicranial recordings render this simple rule more complicated: in humans positive potentials related to cognitive processing occur frequently over parietal regions, especially in tasks which involve the acoustic modality and the processing of perceived and stored information[22,23,26]. The electrophysiological basis of this slow positive shift is unknown. The folding of the cortex could lead to an inversion of the polarity of DC-potentials in scalp electrodes[21]. In particular, activations restricted to a small area located in a cortical sulcus could cause a positivation. In our study, this has to be discussed as a possible cause of left-temporal positivation in the case of activation of the left planum temporale. However, the interindividual variations in polarity are not explained by a theory referring to anatomical facts common to all subjects. It is probable that functional properties related to individual cognitive strategies contribute via inter- and intra-hemispheric inhibitory processes to surface-positive DC-potential shifts.

*Variability and Constancy of Cortical
Activation Patterns*

The considerable interindividual variations in cortical activation are characteristic features of activation patterns obtained in tasks comprising long and complex cognitive operations. The paradigms used in our experiments require decoding of verbal material, access to the mental lexicon, selection of appropriate synonyms, short-time storage of stimulus and synonyms and inner speech. Individual mnemonic strategies and visual associations play a role, factors which are difficult to control since they are not always subject to consciousness. To our opinion, the interindividual variability is the price one has to pay in order to obtain interpretable DC-potentials related to complex neuropsychological functions. Despite the large variations in amplitude, polarity and lateralization, the practically important information remains uniform and clear: fronto-central lateralization of sustained DC-potentials correlates to hemispheric dominance for language. To our knowledge, recording of DC-potentials yields the largest lateralization-effects and thus seems to be a more reliable electrophysiological method assessing speech-dominance than recordings of event related potentials in the shorter latency range from 100 to 600 ms (for a review see[7,24]).

Concerning the intra-individual stability of these findings, we could show in our experiments, that polarity- and lateralization patterns remain stable (negativation or positivation, left- or right-hemispheric lateralization), but may vary in amplitude in two subsequent recordings. This may be due to unspecific effects such as the decrease of attention during the second set of stimuli. In previous experiments with a similar design we investigated the subjects again in a second experimental session one month to one year later and found that activation patterns are stable within a one-year period in adults[1]. In children, however, individual activation patterns change during intellectual development; these changes, which may include the development of new strategies involving different regions of the brain may be due to prolonged learning[4].

Conclusions

Can the WADA-test be replaced by recording of DC-potentials? Our results are encouraging to give a positive answer but prior to a practical application of the DC-method further investigations are necessary. Preoperative assessment of hemispheric dominance in neurosurgery is a very responsible testing since a patient's speech may be severely impaired in case of a false diagnosis. A limitation of our study is the small number of patients so far recruited for external validation. At present, validity and retest-reliability are tested in a larger population of patients with transient as well as persistent impairments of speech. As the most conclusive study, a direct comparison of WADA-test and DC-recordings in patients with chronic, drug-resistant epilepsy is planned.

Compared to alternative methods used to determine hemispheric dominance, recording of DC-potentials has several advantages: It is noninvasive, safe, comparatively inexpensive and can be used repeatedly. For practical application, positioning of frontal electrodes will suffice to determine language dominance. Thus, duration of an examination will be reduced to about 30 minutes, but it should be mentioned that DC-recordings have some methodological limitations: During word-processing, co-operation of the patient is necessary to obtain an appropriate cortical activation and to eliminate artifacts arising from extra-cerebral sources (eye-, tongue-movements, mechanical artifacts from head movements). Sweating artifacts may occasionally pose a problem but can be surmounted by improved recording procedures as proposed recently[5].

To conclude with a more general point of view, analysis of cortical DC-potentials during higher cognitive functions is a promising field in electrophysiology. The topography of activation patterns corresponds to classical localization-theories, based on experiences of neurologists and neurosurgeons. Electrophysiological correlates of individual cognitive strategies can be monitored and classified. In the future, analysis of single trials will provide further insights with respect to the functional organization of cortical networks during cognitive operations and learning processes.

Acknowledgement

The authors wishes to thank Mrs. H. Uhl for experimental assistance and preparation of the figures and Dr. B. Will from the Department of Neurosurgery in Tübingen for the clinical examination and follow up of patient BS.

Appendix

List of stimuli used (translated from German language)

Stimuli with more Abstract Semantical Content

Stimulus	Possible target-words
1. hurry	rush, urgency, scurry
2. state	condition, government
3. form	construct, design, fashion
4. idea	thought, concept
5. stuff	matter, substance, material
6. state	country, nation, territory
7. power	authority, dominance
8. belief	trust, ideology
9. ground	reason, basis
10. search	investigation, inquiry, inspection
11. part	piece, fragment, portion
12. judgment	arbitration, finding, award
13. advice	counsel, guidance
14. mockery	scoffing, ridicule
15. presumption	supposition, hypothesis
16. help	aid, assist, cooperate
17. reproach	reprove, blame
18. commerce	business, trade
19. contract	agreement, deal, pact
20. caution	care, discretion
21. effort	labour, stress
22. thesis	hypothesis, statement
23. talent	ability, genius
24. cunning	crafty, tricky, cleverness
25. law	decree, principle
26. choice	selection, alternative
27. opinion	estimation, impression, mind
28. answer	response, reply
29. proof	evidence, attestation
30. leisure	quiet, relaxation, rest

Stimuli with more Concrete Semantical Content

Stimulus	Possible target-words
1. house	building, home, homestead
2. forest	wood, copse, grove
3. skirt	garment, frock, dress, border
4. dog	bitch, hound, canine
5. tree	sapling, bush, shrub
6. hotel	bed and breakfast, hostel
7. town	city, municipality
8. picture	painting, photograph
9. sofa	couch, divan
10. cord	string, rope, line
11. ship	boat, vessel, barge
12. door	entrance, gate
13. plant	flower, vegetable, herb
14. lamp	light, candle, bulb
15. friend	companion, comrade
16. festivity	festival, celebration
17. fruit	crop
18. vapour	smoke, fog, fumes
19. stair	staircase, steps
20. dam	barrier, mole
21. bed	bedstead, berth, bunk
22. book	album, diary, notebook
23. parcel	bundle, carton, pack
24. meadow	lawn, pasture
25. rock	cliff, crag
26. skin	pelt, coat
27. wing	airfoil, blade, sane
28. river	stream, brook
29. car	motor-vehicle, auto
30. fountain	well, spring

References

1. Altenmüller E (1986) Hirnelektrische Korrelate der cerebralen Musikverarbeitung beim Menschen. Eur Arch Psychiatr Sci 235: 579–587

2. Altenmüller E (1989) Cortical DC-potentials as electrophysiological correlates of hemispheric dominance of higher cognitive functions. Intern J Neuroscience 47: 1–14

3. Altenmüller E, Jung R, Winker T, Landwehrmeyer B (1989) Premotor programming and cortical processing in the cerebral cortex. Brain Behav Evol 33: 141–146

4. Altenmüller E, Kriechbaum W, Baumgärtner R, Moini S (1990) Developmental changes of cortical activation patterns during language and calculation processing: a DC-potential study. In: Brunia CHM et al (eds) Proceedings of the IX Int. Conference on Event-Related Brain Potential Research. Tilburg, Tilburg University Press

5. Bauer H, Korunka C, Leodolter M (1989) Technical requirements for high-quality scalp DC recordings. Electroencephalogr Clin Neurophysiol 72: 545–547

6. Birbaumer N, Lutzenberger W, Elbert T, Rockstroh B, Schwarz J (1981) EEG and slow cortical potentials in anticipation of mental tasks with different hemispheric involvement. Biol Psychol 13: 251–260

7. Brown WS, Marsh JT, Ponsford RE (1987) Hemispheric differences in event-related potentials. In: Benson DF, Zaidel E (eds) The dual brain. Guildford Press, New York, pp 163–179

8. Caspers H, Speckmann EJ, Lehmenkühler A (1984) Electrogenesis of slow potentials of the brain. In: Elbert T et al. (eds) Selfregulation of the brain and behaviour. Springer, Berlin Heidelberg New York, pp 26–41

9. Ely PW, Graves RE, Potter SM (1989) Dichotic listening indices of right hemisphere semantic processing. Neuropsychologia 27: 1007–1015

10. Falconer MA (1971) Anterior temporal lobectomy for epilepsy. In: Logue V (ed) Operative surgery, Vol 14. Butterworths, London, pp 142–149

11. Falconer MA, Serafetinides EA (1963) A follow-up study of surgery in temporal lobe epilepsy. J Neurol Neurosurg Psychiatry 26: 154–165

12. Gevins AS (1987) Correlation analysis. In: Gevins AS, Remond A (eds) Methods of analysis of brain electrical and magnetic signals. EEG Handbook (revised series, Vol 1). Elsevier, Amsterdam, pp 171–193

13. Goodglass H, Klein B, Carey P, Jones K (1966) Specific semantic word categories in aphasia. Cortex 2: 74–89

14. Heiss WD, Herholz K, Pawlik G, Wagner R, Wienhard K (1986) Positron emission tomography in neuropsychology. Neuropsychologia 24: 141–149

15. Ingvar DH (1983) Serial aspects of language and speech related to prefrontal cortical activity. A selective review. Human Neurobiol 2: 177–189

16. Jung R, Altenmüller E, Natsch B (1984) Zur Hemisphärendominanz für Sprache und Rechnen: Elektrophysiologische Korrelate einer Linksdominanz bei Linkshändern. Neuropsychologia 22: 755–775

17. Mateer CA, Dodrill CB (1983) Neuropsychological and linguistic correlates of atypical language lateralization: Evidence from sodium amytal studies. Human Neurobiol 2: 135–142

18. Oldfield RC (1971) The assessment and analysis of handedness: the Edinburgh inventory. Neuropsychologia 9: 97–113

19. Rassmussen T, Millner B (1977) The role of early left-brain injury in determining lateralization of cerebral speech functions. Ann NY Acad Sci 299: 355–369

20. Risberg J (1986) Regional cerebral blood flow in neuropsychology. Neuropsychologia 24: 135–140

21. Rockstroh B, Elbert T, Canavan A, Lutzenberger W, Birbaumer N (1990) Slow brain potentials and behaviour (second edition). Urban Schwarzenberg, München, pp 85–125

22. Rösler F, Clausen G, Sojka B (1986) The double-priming paradigma: a tool for analyzing the functional significance of endogenous event-related brain potentials. Biol Psychology 22: 239–268

23. Ruchkin DS, Sutton S (1983) Positive slow wave and P300: association and disassociation. In: Gaillard AW et al. (eds) Tutorials in Event-Related potential research: endogenous components. Elsevier, Amsterdam, pp 233–250

24. Rugg M, Kok A, Barett G, Fischler I (1986) ERPs associated with language and hemispheric specialization. A review. In: McCallum WC et al (eds) Cerebral psychophysiology: Studies in event-related potentials. Elsevier, Amsterdam, pp 273–299

25. Shaw JC, O'Connor K, Ongley C (1978) EEG Coherence as a measure of cerebral functional organisation. In: Brazier MAB, Petsche H (eds) Architectonics of the cerebral cortex. Raven Press, New York, pp 245–255

26. Sutton S, Ruchkin DS (1984) The late positive complex: Advances and new problems. In: Karrer R et al.(eds) Brain and information: Event related potentials. Ann NY Acad Sci, pp 1–23

27. Wada J (1949) A new method for the determination of the side of cerebral speech dominance: A preliminary report on the intracarotid injection of sodium amytal in man. Igaku to Seibutsugako 14: 221–222

28. Wada J, Rasmussen T (1960) Intracarotid injection of sodium amytal for the lateralization of cerebral speech dominance. J Neurosurg 17: 266–282

29. Warrington EK, Shallice T (1984) Category specific semantic impairments. Brain 107: 829–854

Correspondence: E. Altenmüller, Department of Neurology, University of Tübingen, Hoppe-Seyler-Str. 3, 7, D-W-7400 Tübingen, Federal Republic of Germany.

Acta Neurochirurgica (1993) [Suppl] 56: 34–39

Brain Mapping in Thinking and Language Function

L. Friberg

Department of Clinical Physiology & Nuclear Medicine, Glostrup Hospital, Copenhagen, Denmark

Summary

Regional cerebral blood flow, rCBF, is coupled to regional cerebral metabolism and changes in rCBF reflects changes in neuronal activity. rCBF studies have provided information about the functions of a great number of cortical regions in the normal human brain. Outside the motor areas and sensory association areas there are areas committed to the transformation of information retrieved or generated within the brain itself. Language is processed within these regions. In contrast to the general clinical impression the functional mapping methods reveal that there is a large number of cortical regions activated bilaterally during language processing. Pure intrinsic brain work causes a profound activation of the cerebral cortex. Different types of thinking are seen to activate different sectors of the cortical space.

Keywords: Regional cerebral blood flow; language processing regions; brain mapping.

Introduction

A century ago Roy and Sherrington (1890) suggested that cerebral blood flow would increase during neuronal activity and that this increase was related to an increased metabolic rate in the brain. Fulton (1928) reported that in a patient with an arteriovenous malformation in the occipital lobe there was an increased bruit over the scalp as soon as he opened his eyes, which supported the hypothesis of Roy and Sherrington. Moreover, the bruit increased further when the patient was reading. It was not until 1948 it became possible to measure the actual blood flow and oxygen consumption in the human brain[17]. With the Kety–Schmidt technique global blood flow and global metabolism could be measured (Kety 1950). The sensitivity of this method was, however, not sufficient to detect changes in the total cerebral blood flow or metabolism during physiological activation, e.g. during mental brain work[45]. With the regional cerebral blood flow, rCBF, method introduced by Lassen and Ingvar (1961,

1963)[19,20], it became possible to measure changes in blood flow in fairly small cortical regions; for example when a subject was speaking[13] or was moving his hand[32]. In the normal human brain, the rCBF is coupled to the regional cerebral oxygen consumption[21,24,36,41]. There is also a close temporal correlation between the onset and termination of increased neuronal impulse frequency and the increased rCBF[28]. Therefore, during physiologically normal conditions blood flow changes in small cortical regions are an indirect way of detecting the neuronal activity in these regions. As spatial resolution gradually improved, the rCBF equipment was refined and further developed into single photon emission tomography, SPECT, it became possible to perform functional mapping studies of the human cerebral cortex. The positron emission tomography, PET, technique was introduced. With PET it is possible to perform functional mapping of the brain by measuring both rCBF, regional metabolic rate of oxygen and regional metabolic rate of glucose[10,21,27,38,41].

This review will focus on the methods used and findings from studies of cortical activity during complex language processing and during pure mental activity. It will mainly summarize some rCBF studies, as rCBF is a rapidly obtainable and reliable parameter for functional brain mapping studies both with PET, SPECT and other types of equipment.

Considerations on Method

The *Kety–Schmidt technique* (1948) was based on the principles of Fick (1870) and implied simultaneous sampling of blood from the carotid artery and the jugular vein after 10 min of inhalation of the inert gas nitrous oxide. By measuring the N_2O concentrations in the blood samples Kety and Schmidt obtained a mean value of whole brain blood flow of 54 ± 12 ml/100 g/min in a group of 14 young, healthy and conscious subjects. They also calculated values for cerebral O_2 consumption. The method is very exact for determination of whole brain blood flow but not sensitive to focal CBF changes[45].

The Intra-carotid Xe-133 Injection Technique

With the intra-carotid Xe-133 injection technique rCBF is usually measured in direct connection with performance of a cerebral angiography. After puncture of one of the common carotid arteries a thin soft polyethylene catheter is introduced into the internal carotid artery (using the Seldinger technique. Xe-133 dissolved in saline is injected through the catheter and for the following 2 minutes the clearance of isotope is recorded with a 254 multidetector gamma camera covering one hemisphere[47]. For each detector rCBF is calculated from 12–60 seconds after the bolus injection[33]. Usually there is a time interval of 10 minutes between each measurement and 6 to 8 further measurements can be obtained during one session. The intra-carotid method is very precise in respect to measuring exact flow values in grey matter and has become the "golden" standard for measurements of rCBF. Unfortunately the method is traumatic and it is now only used in the examination of a few selected patients in whom there is indication for direct carotid puncture for the purpose of performing angiography or Wada-test[40].

Furthermore the method does not allow examination of both hemispheres simultaneously.

Stationary Detector Systems and Xe-133

rCBF is measured with 32 and up to 254 detectors covering both hemispheres. Xe-133 can be injected i.v. or inhaled. rCBF can be calculated either from a two-compartmental analysis[31,35] or as the Initial Slope Index, ISI[37].

SPECT and Xe-133 Inhalation

As arrival to and washout of Xe-133 from the brain is a fast dynamic process the SPECT equipment for measurements of rCBF has to be highly sensitive and brain dedicated[3,23,46], (Lassen and Friberg 1988). The Tomomatic SPECT systems can measure rCBF in 2–5 slices simultaneously the slices usually are positioned parallel to the orbitometal plane. Each slice is 17 mm thick and the distance between the center-line of each slice is 40 mm. The resolution is down 12 mm in the transverse plane. One study lasts 4.5 minutes. There must be an interval of at least 25 minutes between each measurement – enabling the Xe-133 to be washed out – in order to ensure reasonably low residual activity in the brain before further studies.

SPECT Retained rCBF Tracers: Tc-99 m-HMPAO

By changing the lead collimators in front of the crystals and using a retained type of radio-labelled flow tracer the resolution of this type of equipment can be increased down to 8–10 mm. A conventional rotating Anger gamma camera can also be used in connection with the retained isotopes[4]. A two or three headed modification of this camera can provide a resolution of approximately 10 mm[15]. After intravenous injection of the lipophilic Tc-99 m-HMPAO the compound is circulated with the blood to the brain. The compound immediately diffuses into the cells of the brain, where almost instantly it is converted to a hydrophillic substances which is trapped within the brain during the first minute after injection. The distribution of trapped Tc-99 m-HMPAO represents the blood flow distribution following the first minute after injection[1,22,29]. It is possible to administer two doses of Tc-99 m-HMPAO with short

intervals and in this way study pharmacological or physiological induced relative rCBF changes within the brain. It is recommended to use about 1/3 of the total dose for the first injection. After the first scanning session the picture obtained can be used as background for the second picture. The second picture can be obtained after a subsequent injection of the remaining 2/3 of the dose[11,44]. This procedure will ensure approximately the same statistics on count rates. The technique is at present undergoing further development in our laboratories with the purpose of using Tc-99 m-HMPAO during activation studies.

Mapping of Language Function

Figure 1 illustrates that only a minor part of the human cerebral cortex is predetermined to primary handling of incoming information or to the execution of voluntary movements. Most of the frontal lobes and large parts of the parietal and temporal lobes are not selectively devoted to sensory or motor functions. These regions comprise the so-called uncommitted cortex (Penfield 1966). However, the term uncommitted does not imply that these cortex regions are unspecialized or unorganized. The cortical activation patterns seen during language processing and speech are examples of how some higher intellectual functions,

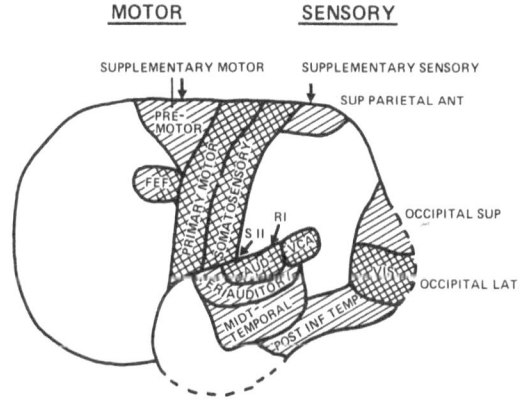

☒ Primary motor and sensory zones (+ immediate sensory areas)
☒ Premotor areas and intermediate + remote sensory areas.
☐ Uncommitted cortex.

Fig. 1. Motor and sensory areas of the human cerebral cortex based on functional mapping studies carried out with rCBF methods. The primary sensory areas are surrounded by immediate, intermediate and remote association areas. The secondary somatosensory area (*SII*) and the retroinsular cortex (*RI*) are only visible with three dimensional methods. With the two dimensional rCBF methods the primary auditory cortex in the lateral sulcus is recorded in a tangential view. This area was always co-activated with the surrounding immediate association cortex (*AUD*). The activation of the vestibular cortical area (*VCA*) was not associated with rCBF increases in other cortical regions with the two dimensional method (Friberg *et al.* 1985). rCBF increases have been recorded from the frontal eye fields (*FEF*) both during motor and sensory tasks. The white areas of the figure illustrate the large extension of the uncommitted cortex regions (Penfield 1966)

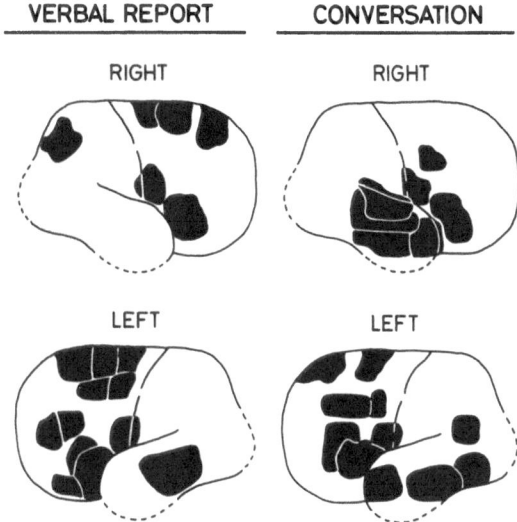

VERBAL REPORT   CONVERSATION

RIGHT   RIGHT

LEFT   LEFT

Fig. 2. The average outline and location of the areas activated during verbal report from visual memory and during conversation. In the black areas rCBF increased significantly. The figure illustrates the bilateral involvement of the hemisphere, despite all the subjects being considered to be left hemispheric dominant for the language function

unique for man, have the participation cortical fields localized to regions within the uncommitted cortex. rCBF changes have been studied during discrimination of tonal patterns[34], during listening to simple words[14,18], during simple (automatic) speech[30], when speaking fluently and conversing (Friberg *et al.* 1987) and when reading[14,18]. These and other studies have provided information on how relatively simple language tasks activated the cortex (for review see Ingvar 1983).

Figure 2 shows the patterns of cortical areas activated during two different kinds of complex linguistic brain work (Friberg and Roland 1988). The subjects of these studies were all strictly right-handed and during the rCBF measurements their eyes were closed and covered. During verbal report from visual memory the subjects had to describe fluently a spatially arranged, finite number of well-known objects: every piece of furniture in their living room.

In the second study the subjects conversed with the examiner on the topic: How do you usually spend Christmas Eve? The subjects were requested to answer in fluent speech with as accurate descriptions as possible, but were regularly interrupted when the examiner asked new questions. In the activated regions there were statistically significant rCBF increases from 9 to 30%. Both tasks increased rCBF in the visual association areas: the posterior superior parietal cortex and the posterior inferior temporal cortex. It has been suggested that visual memories could be represented in these areas (Roland and Friberg 1985). Furthermore

there was activation of the superior prefrontal cortex during both tasks, most likely because these areas participate in organization of brain work in general (Roland and Friberg 1985). The mid-temporal areas and the posterior inferior frontal areas, which are the Broca area in the left hemisphere and Broca's homologue in the right hemisphere, were activated bilaterally, presumably due to their participation in retrieval of names and production of sentences.

It is interesting to note that Broca's area and Broca's right-sided homologue were not found significantly activated during automatic speech[18]. This indicates that involvement of these areas is not necessarily required when performing simple, almost reflex-like, linguistic tasks as when reciting the days of the week or when counting repeatedly to twenty[18]. In both the verbal report task and the conversation task the actually spoken words were requested and the motor component of speech was reflected by activation of the supplementary motor areas and the primary motor area of the mouth. When the subjects were conversing and listened to the examiners questions, the right auditory and periauditory areas were activated. But when they spoke without interruption, there was surprisingly no rCBF increase in these areas in any of the two hemispheres. This might indicate that the subjects were not paying more attention to their own speech than to the almost abolished auditory input during the resting condition[7]. Additionally the conversation task activated the frontal eye field bilaterally, probably provoked by the attention payed to the external auditory stimulus. During both tasks there was activation of several mid- and inferior prefrontal areas in the left hemisphere. Activation of these areas is seen during different kinds of mental brain work and it was not possible to relate the activation of these areas to language spoken or received.

Although all the subjects could be considered left hemisphere dominant for language, the rCBF studies have shown that there is a high degree of involvement of symmetrically located areas in both hemispheres during different language tasks[8,26].

Normal function of the language areas of the dominant hemisphere, described by Broca (1861) and Wernicke (1874), is vital for normal language processing, but they are by far the only cortical areas involved in linguistic brain work. It has been suggested that the cortical activity associated with language and speech is controlled by serial mechanisms (Ingvar 1983).

During listening to simple words[30] and when performing automatic speech the numbers of activated cortical areas were less and the rCBF increases in the activated areas smaller than when subjects were speaking fluently or conversing[40]. Therefore, simple enumeration or listening to simple words or sounds can be considered part-functions of the language used during fluent speech or conversation.

Pure Intrinsic Brain Work: Thinking

Roland and Friberg (1985) studied three different kinds of brain work, in the form of operations on internal information; these were done by awake subjects. They were completely silent, the eyes and ears were covered, they did not receive any sensory stimulation and they did not execute voluntary movements. Before each measurement the subjects were carefully instructed and

trained to solve thinking tasks similar to those performed during the actual rCBF measurement.

During numerical operation the subjects were asked, internally to subtract 3 from 50 and then 3 from the result and so on for the whole 48 second period of measurement. After termination of the rCBF measurement they were asked what result they had reached. During jingle thinking the subjects were asked, inside their brains, to recite a well known Danish jingle. Every second word of this closed-loop jingle was internally recited over and over. During route finding the subjects were asked to imagine that they walked in well-known surroundings: the streets around their homes. They started at their front door, then they imagined walking to the left, then down the first street to the right and then they imagined that they walked alternatively to

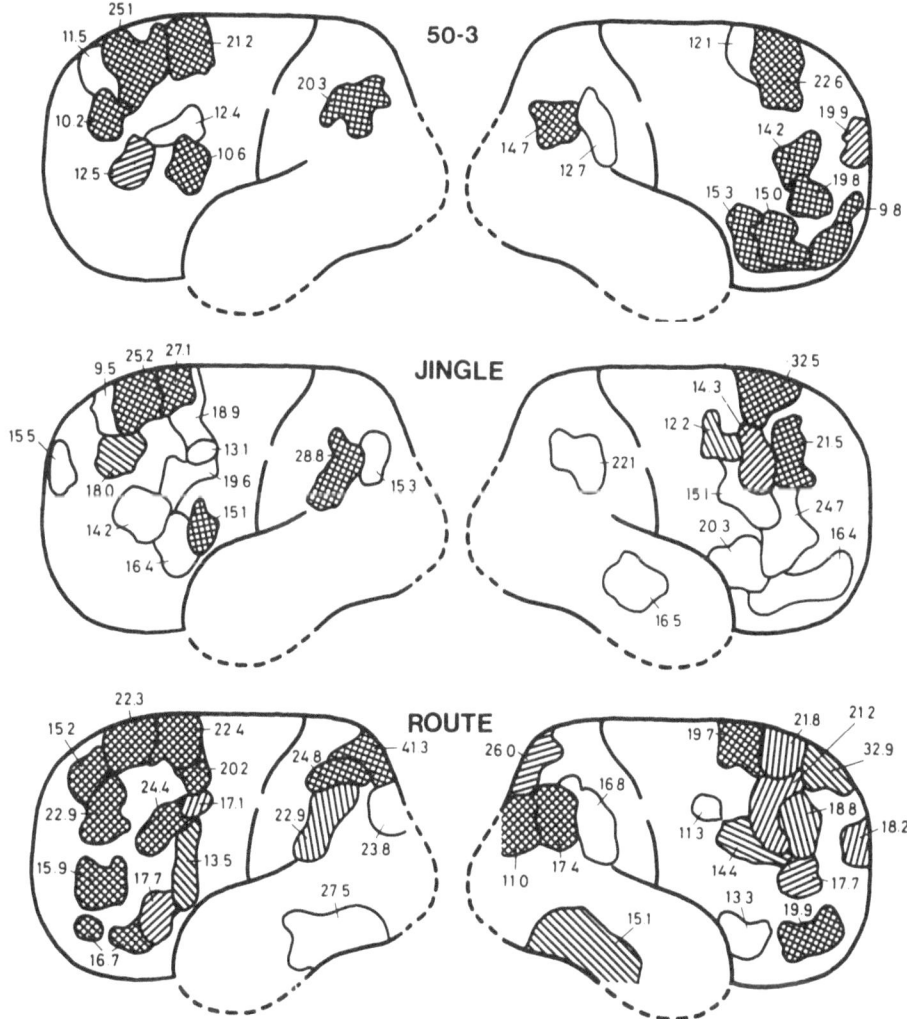

Fig. 3. Mean percentage increases of rCBF and their average distribution in the cerebral cortex during three different types of thinking. Left = left hemisphere. Right = right hemisphere. In cross-hatched areas the rCBF increases were statistically significant at the 0.005 level (t-test, two sided comparison). Hatched areas $P < 0.01$ and other areas $P < 0.05$. Note that only the cortex outside the motor and sensory areas was activated and that no significant decreases in rCBF were observed. (From Roland and Friberg 1985 with permission)

the left and the right every time they reached a corner. They were told not to try to remember names of streets or buildings, but were asked to recall the surroundings visually only.

These three types of thinking produced three different patterns of multifocal significant rCBF increases (Fig. 3). Thinking was mainly produced in homotypical areas within the uncommitted cortex and there was complete lack of activation of the motor zones and of the primary and immediate sensory zones. There was, however, activation of the remote auditory association areas during jingle thinking and activation of the remote visual association areas during the route-finding task. The Broca area and Broca's right-sided homologue were activated during all tasks, perhaps indicating that some form of internal speech was processed during thinking. The estimated cortical energy consumption during thinking was equivalent to or larger than the estimated cortical energy consumption during voluntary movements or when processing external sensory stimulation[40].

References

1. Andersen AR, Friberg HH, Schmidt JF, Hasselbalch SG (1988) Quantitative measurements of cerebral blood flow using SPECT and 99 m-Tc-d, IHM-PAO compared to Xenon-313. J Cereb Blood Flow Metab 8: 69–81

2. Broca PP (1861) Remarques sur le siège de la faculté du language articulé. Bull Soc d'antropol 33: 330–336

3. Celsis P, Goldman T, Henriksen L, Lassen NA (1981) A method for calculating regional cerebral blood flow from emission computed tomography of inert gas concentrations. J Comput Assist Tomogr 5: 641–645

4. English RE, Holman L (1987) Current status of cerebral perfusion radiopharmaceuticals. J Nucl Med Technol 15: 30

5. Fick A (1870) Über die Messung des Blutquantums in den Herzventrikeln. Ver Phys Med Ges Würzburg 2: 16

6. Friberg L, Skyhøj Olsen T, Roland PE, Paulson OB, Lassen NA (1985) Focal increase of blood flow in the cerebral cortex of man during vestibular stimulation. Brain 108: 609–623

7. Friberg L, Roland PE (1988) Functional activation and inhibition of regional cerebral blood flow and metabolism. In: Olesen J, Edvinsson L (eds) Basic mechanisms of headache. Elsevir, pp. 89–98

8. Friberg L, Lassen NA (1991) Language and the cerebral hemispheres: Impact of stimulus relevance and absence of lateralized activation response as revealed by rCBF studies. In: Lassen NA, Ingvar DH, Raichle ME, Friberg L (eds). Brain Work and Mental Activity. Munksgaard, Copenhagen-Chicago-Tokyo, pp 294–308

9. Fulton JF (1928) Observations upon vascularity of the human occipital lobe during visual activity. Brain 51: 310–320

10. Ginsberg MD, Howard BE, Hassel WR (1984) Emission tomography measurement of local cerebral blood flow in humans by an in vivo autoradiographic strategy. Ann Neurol 15 [Suppl]: 12–18

11. Holm S, Madsen PL, Rubin P, Sperling B, Friberg L, Lassen NA (1991) Tc-99m-HMPAO activation studies: Validation of split-lose, image subtraction approach. J Cereb Blood Flow Metab 11 (Suppl. 2): 5766

12. Ingvar DH (1983) Serial aspects of language and speech related to prefrontal cortical activity. Human Neurobiology 2: 177–189

13. Ingvar DH, Risberg J (1967) Increase of regional cerebral blood flow during mental effort in normals and in patients with focal brain disorders. Exp Brain Res 3: 195–211

14. Ingvar DH, Schwartz MS (1974) Blood flow patterns induced in the dominant hemisphere by speech and reading. Brain 97: 273–288

15. Jaszczak RJ, Coleman RE (1988) Instrumentation for single-photon computed tomography studies of the brain. Am J Physiol Imaging 3: 67

16. Kety SS (1950) Circulation and metabolism of the human brain in health and disease. Am J Med 8: 205–217

17. Kety SS, Schmidt CFS (1948) The nitrous oxide method for the quantitative determination of cerebral blood flow in man. Theory, procedure and normal values. J Clin Invest 27: 476–483

18. Larsen B, Skinhøj E, Lassen NA (1978) Variations in regional cortical blood flow in the right and left hemispheres during automatic speech. Brain 101: 193–209

19. Lassen NA, Ingvar DH (1961) The blood flow of the cerebral cortex determined by radioactive Crypton-85. Experienta 17: 42–43

20. Lassen NA, Ingvar DH (1963) Regional cerebral blood flow measurements in man. Arch Neurol Psychiat 9: 615–622

21. Lassen NA, Ingvar DH, Raichle ME, Friberg L (1991) Brain Work and Mental Activity. Quantitative studies with radioactive tracers. Munksgaard, Copenhagen-Chicago-Tokyo, pp 1–445

22. Lassen NA, Andersen AR, Friberg L, Paulson OB (1988) The retention of 99 m-Tc-d, IHM-PAO in human brain after intracarotid bolus injection: A kinetic analysis. J. Cereb Blood Flow Metab 8: 13–22

23. Lassen NA, Sveinsdottir E, Kanno I, Stokely EM, Rommer P (1978) A fast rotating single photon emission tomograph for regional cerebral blood flow studies in man. J Comput Assist Tomogr 2: 660–661

24. Lebrun-Grandié P, Baron J-C, Soussaline F, Loch'h C, Sastre J, Bousser M-G (1983) Coupling between regional cerebral blood flow and oxygen utilization in the normal human brain. Arch Neurol 40: 230–236

25. Madsen PL, Schmidt JF, Holm S, Jorgersen H, Wildschiødtz, Christensen NJ, Friberg L, Vorstrap S, Lassen NA (1992) Mental Stress and Cogretive performance do not increase overall level of cerebral O_2. Update in humans. J Appl Physiol 73: 420–426

26. Mchaughlin T, Steinberg B, Christensen B, Law I, Parving A, Friberg L (1992) Potential language and attentional networks revealed through factor analysis of rCBF data. J Cereb Blood Flow Metab 12: 335–345

27. Mazziotta JC, Phelps ME (1984) Human sensory stimulation and deprivation: Positron emission tomographic results and strategies. Ann Neurol 15 [Suppl]: 50–60.

28. Moskalenko YY (1975) Regional cerebral blood flow and its control at rest and during increased functional activity. In: Ingvar DH, Lassen Na (eds) Brain work. Munksgaard, Copenhagen, pp 343–351

29. Neirinckx RD, Burke JF, Harrison RC, Forster AM, Andersen AR, Lassen NA (1988) The retention mechanism of technetium-99 m-HM-PAO: Intracellular reaction with glutathione. J Cereb Blood Flow Metab 8: 4–12

30. Nishizawa Y, Olsen TS, Larsen B, Lassen NA (1982) Left-right cortical asymmetries of regional cerebral blood flow during listening to words. J Neurophysiol 48: 458–466

31. Obrist WD, Thompson HK, Wang HS, Wilkinson WE (1975) Regional cerebral blood flow estimated by Xenon-133 inhalation. Stroke 6: 245–256

32. Olesen J (1971) Contralateral focal increase of cerebral blood flow in man during arm work. Brain 94: 635–646

33. Olesen J, Paulson OB, Lassen NA (1971) Regional cerebral blood flow in man determined by initial slope of intra-arterially injected Xe-133. Stroke 2: 519–540

34. Penfield W (1966) Speech, perception and the uncommitted cortex. In: Eccels JC (ed) Brain and conscious experience. Springer, Berlin Heidelberg New York, pp 217–237

35. Prohovnik I, Knudsen E, Risberg J (1983) Accuracy of models and algorithms for determination of fast component flow by non-invasive Xenon-133 clearance. In: Magistretti PL (ed) Functional radionucleide imaging of the brain. Raven Press, New York, pp 97–115

36. Raichle ME, Grubb RL, Gado MH, Eichling JO, Ter-Pogossian MM (1976) Correlation between regional cerebral blood flow and oxidative metabolism. Arch Neurol 33: 523–526

37. Risberg J, Ali Z, Wilson EM, Wills EL, Halsey JH (1975) Regional cerebral blood flow by Xenon-133 inhalation. Preliminary evaluation of an initial slope index in patients with unstable flow compartments. Stroke 6: 142–148

38. Roland PE (1982) Cortical regulation of selective attention in man. J Neurophysiol 48: 1059–1078

39. Roland PE, Skinhøj E, Lassen NA (1981) Focal activations of the human cerebral cortex during auditory discrimination. J Neurophysiol 45: 374–386

40. Roland PE, Friberg L (1985) Localization of cortical areas activated by thinking. J Neurophysiol 53: 1219–1243

41. Roland PE, Eriksson L, Stone-Elander S, Widen L (1987) Increases of regional cerebral oxidative metabolism and regional cerebral blood flow provoked by visual imagery. J Neurosci 7: 2373

42. Roland PE, Friberg L (1988) The effect of the GABA-A agonist THIP on regional cortical blood flow in humans. A new test of hemispheric dominance. J Cereb Blood Flow Metab 8: 314–323

43. Roy CS, Sherrington CS (1890) On regulation of the blood supply of the brain. J Physiol (London) 11: 85–108

44. Rubin P, Holm S, Friberg L, Videbuk P, Andersen HS, Berg-Bertsen B, Strømsø N, Lassen NA, Hemmingsen R (1991) Altered modulation of prefrontal and subcortical brain activity in newly diagnosed schizophreria and schizo-phreriform disorder: A regional cerebral blood flow study. Arch Gen Psychiat 48: 987–995

45. Sokoloff L, Mangold R, Wechsler RL, Kennedy C, Kety SS (1955) The effect of mental arithmetic on cerebral circulation and metabolism. J Clin Invest 34: 1101–1108

46. Stokely EM, Sveinsdottir E, Lassen NA, Rommer P (1980) A single photon dynamic computer-assisted tomograph (DCAT) for imaging brain function in multiple cross-sections. J Comput Assist Tomogr 4: 142–148

47. Sveinsdottir E, Larsen B, Rommer P, Lassen NA (1977) A multidetector scintillation camera with 254 channels. J Nucl Med 18: 168–174

48. Wernicke C (1874) Der aphasische Symptomenkomplex. Cohn und Weigart, Breslau

Correspondence: L. Friberg, Department of Clinical Physiology and Nuclear Medicine, Glostrup Hospital DK-2600 Glostrup, Denmark.

Acta Neurochirurgica (1993) [Suppl] 56: 40–51

The Effects of Electrostimulation and of Resective and Stereotactic Surgery on Language and Speech

Y. Lebrun and **C. Leleux**

Neurolinguistics, Vrije Universiteit, Brussels, Belgium

Summary

A fairly comprehensive survey is offered of the effects which cortical and sub-cortical electrical stimulation have on language and speech. A survey is also given of the verbal consequences of resections or coagulations which generally follow electrical stimulation.

Keywords: Brain electrostimulation, stereotaxy, language.

Introduction

In an effort to alleviate medically intractable focal epilepsy, neurosurgeons may decide to excise a limited portion of the cerebral cortex together with some of the underlying white matter. Operations of this type are usually preceded by electrical stimulation of the area where the excision is to take place. An electric current is applied to various sites in this area, primarily with a view to finding where it interferes with verbal processes. During the resection, the neurosurgeon as far as possible avoids encroaching upon the sites where interference has been observed.

Another type of neurosurgical intervention which is often preceded by electrostimulation is stereotaxy. Before destroying a sub-cortical structure, the operator frequently stimulates it electrically in an effort to anticipate the results and consequences of the coagulation.

In the present paper, a general survey is offered of the observations made during electrostimulation of the cortex or of sub-cortical structures, and its bearing on verbal behaviour. A survey is also presented of the linguistic deficits which may occur after resective or stereotaxic surgery.

Electrostimulation

1. Cortical Stimulation

At times electrostimulation of the cortex takes place intra-operatively. In this procedure, craniotomy is performed under local anaesthesia. Then a current is applied successively at various sites in the exposed cortex and the effects of stimulation are recorded. The patient remains conscious throughout the procedure.

In other cases chronic subdural electrodes are placed under general anaesthesia and stimulation is performed extra-operatively.

Electrostimulation of the cortex in conscious individuals may result in two different types of neurolinguistic conditions. The experimental excitation may cause the subject to produce sounds involuntarily or it may interfere with the verbal activity the subject is performing.

Involuntary Vocalization

Involuntary vocalization as a result of electrical stimulation of the precentral cortex was initially described by Penfield (1938)[28]. A continuous, even vowel sound was elicited from various points in the face subdivision of the motor area. The response continued for the duration of stimulation or until maximum expiration was reached. Then there was a pause for breathing, after which the sound was resumed.

The patients were aware of their vocalizations but could not suppress them. One patient said to the surgeon at the end of a stimulation that had caused loud vocalization: "It felt as though you were pulling the voice out of me".

Involuntary vocalization could be observed during stimulation of the left as well as of the right hemisphere.

A different kind of vocal response elicited from the mesial surface of the frontal lobe anterior to the leg subdivision of the motor strip, was originally reported by Brickner (1940)[5]. His patient vocalized in a repetitive manner upon electrical stimulation.

This type of intermittent vocalization was also observed by Penfield and Welch (1951)[30] upon stimulation of the same area. The sound produced repetitively could be a vowel or a syllable.

However, at times electrical excitation of the supplementary motor area elicited an exclamation or a prolonged vowel sound. Periodic changes in pitch and volume gave some protracted sounds a rhythmic character. Others of the sustained vocalizations showed gradual elevation of pitch and reduction of volume.

Associated with these vocal responses were sometimes seen facial movements involving both sides of the mouth and the jaw. These movements were often homorhythmic with the periodic variations in volume of the sound or with each sound in an intermittent vocalization.

Such reactions could be obtained from both cerebral hemispheres. Patients who were asked why they had produced sounds under electrical stimulation said that they could not help it.

In one particular patient, whose right post-central and pre-central gyri had been surgically removed in an effort to relieve causalgia-like pain in the paralyzed left side of the body, Penfield and Welch (1951)[30] observed involuntary production of variegated but meaningless syllables during stimulation of the right supplementary motor area.

In sum, electrical stimulation of the mouth area of the motor cortex in either hemisphere may result in the involuntary production of a sustained, even vowel sound, whereas electrical stimulation of the supplementary area may provoke a sustained or intermittent sound possibly accompanied by mouth or jaw movements.

Speech Arrests

In patients who are speaking when the current is applied, stimulation may interfere with speech. The interference may take several forms. At times, a speech arrest is observed, that is to say that the patient is rendered mute by the stimulation. Upon cessation of the current or a little thereafter he is generally able to resume his speaking activity at the point of interruption. For instance, if he is counting when stimulation is applied, there may be a break in the recitation that lasts as long as the stimulus is applied. After withdrawal of the stimulus, counting is resumed.

Walter[7] noted that the patient may at times deny having stopped during stimulation. It is as if the current causes "a sort of time slip" together with the speech arrest.

Under electrical stimulation patients may also be unable to answer questions or to name the objects they are shown. The speech arrest may last longer than the stimulation. During the speech arrest there may be movements of the jaw as if the patient is trying to speak.

If the subject is asked questions during a speech arrest, he may be able to reproduce or answer them once the arrest is over. A patient of Penfield and Welch (1951)[30] in whom stimulation caused a speech arrest, said afterwards to the physician: "I could hear what you were saying, doctor. I knew what I wanted to say, but I just couldn't".

Lesser et al. (1984)[15] found that during an electrically provoked speech arrest the patient may or may not be able to write or to perform rapid alternating movements with his tongue.

Arrests of speech were observed by Penfield and Roberts (1959)[29] following stimulation of the posterior half of the frontal lobe, the banks of the Sylvian fissure and the posterior two-thirds of the second temporal gyrus of the left hemisphere, as well as of the lower half of the precentral and postcentral gyri of the right hemisphere.

Thus, electrical stimulation of the lower half of the precentral and postcentral convolutions and of the supplementary motor area may have both excitatory and inhibitory effects on speech.

On the other hand, the effect of electrical stimulation may be inconstant. For instance, in a case reported by Ojemann and Whitaker (1978)[27] the same frontal site was stimulated five times during an oral naming task. Three times there was a speech arrest, and two times the current did not interfere with speech production. In a patient described by Rapport et al. (1983)[31] five sites were identified at which stimulation inconsistently caused mutism during a naming task and no interference at all during oral reading.

Writing Arrest

If the patient is writing when the current is applied, stimulation may make it impossible for him to continue writing. He is usually able to resume his writing task upon cessation of the current. During a writing arrest, the patient, according to Lesser et al. (1984)[15], may or may not be able to speak. Thus, speech and writing arrests may or may not coincide.

Speech Alterations

At times the electrical stimulus does not suppress speech but alters it. The patient slows down or hesitates or speaks in a faint voice.

Under electrical stimulation patients may also involuntarily iterate words. For instance, the patient of Brickner (1940)[5] could be caused to repeat letters by applying the stimulus while she was reciting the alphabet, and a patient of Penfield and Welch (1951)[30], who was stimulated while he was counting, repeated the "3" for a considerable period.

Stimulation may also result in the substitution of a prolonged or intermittent vocalization for the intended words.

Hesitations, slurring and iterations could be elicited by stimulation of the posterior half of the frontal lobe and the peri-Sylvian area of the left hemisphere, as well as by stimulation of a zone centered around the Rolandic fissure in the right hemisphere[29].

Aphasic Disorders

If stimulation is applied while the patient is performing an oral naming task, the current may prevent him from saying the target word whilst he remains able to speak, that is to say that the electric stimulation may cause anomia.

It may also happen that the patient makes paraphasias, i.e. misnames the objects or pictures shown. The paraphasia may be a perseveration, i.e. the substitution of a previous answer for the present answer.

The sites where the current was observed by Penfield and Roberts (1959)[29], Fedio and Van Buren (1974)[8], Whitaker and Ojemann (1977)[42], Van Buren et al. (1978)[41], Ojemann (1979)[22], Ojemann et al. (1989)[26] to produce anomia, paraphasias, or perseverations were located in the posterior half of the frontal lobe, the banks of the Sylvian fissure, and the posterior two-thirds of the middle temporal gyrus, usually in the left hemisphere.

Ojemann and his colleagues noted that these sites did not form a continuous zone in any single patient. Rather, they were frequently separated by sites where the current did not cause any naming impairment. For instance, in one case, Ojemann and Whitaker (1978)[27] stimulated three different sites all on the same convolution and within 2 cm of each other. At one site, there were 100% naming errors, while there was no error at all at the other two sites. Again, there were frequently sites where the interference was inconstant. The inconsistency in the effects of electrical stimulation

was thought by Whitaker and Ojemann (1977)[42] to reflect a "graded localization of naming functions" in the cerebral cortex.

In a case reported by Fedio and van Buren (1974)[8] there were found, intermingled with sites where naming was disturbed and sites where it was not, loci where naming was correct but where the latency of the response was unusually long.

Ojemann et al. (1989)[26] furthermore observed vast differences in the distribution of the sites where stimulation interfered with oral naming. They concluded that "neither the location nor absence of language function at a given cortical site can be reliably predicted by anatomical considerations". There may be one exception, however. Ojemann and Whitaker (1978)[27], Ojemann (1979)[22] and Lesser et al. (1984)[15] pointed out that in each of their patients electric stimulation of a small portion of the third frontal convolution immediately in front of the left motor strip consistently interfered with speech production.

Occasionally naming could be disturbed by electrostimulation of a site outside the fronto-parieto-temporal zone delineated above. For instance, stimulation of the anterior part of the left temporal lobe by Ojemann et al. (1989)[26] and of the left parieto-temporo-occipital junction by Van Buren et al. (1978)[41] at times resulted in aphasic disturbances.

Disturbances of Verbal Memory

Fedio and Van Buren (1974)[8] found that electrical stimulation of the left temporal and temporo-parietal area may impair short term verbal memory, preventing the patient from recalling the verbal response he gave a few seconds earlier.

In summary, then, investigations using electrostimulation have resulted in the mapping of a fairly large fronto-parieto-temporal area, generally in the left hemisphere, where electric current can interfere with speech and language processes. Stimulation may result in the involuntary production of isolated sounds, which can be prolonged or intermittent, or it may prevent the patient from speaking, or make him repeat or stutter or speak in a slurred way, or it may impair word finding and word selection. It may also disturb short term verbal memory.

Vocalizations, speech arrests and speech alterations can also be caused by electrostimulation of an area in the right hemisphere centered around the rolandic fissure and including the supplementary motor area.

However, not every site within the areas which have

Table 1. *Cortical Electrostimulation*

Sites in the left hemisphere	Verbal behaviours	Sites in the right hemisphere
Lower precentral cortex	Involuntary vocalizations	Lower precentral cortex
Supplementary motor area		Supplementary motor area
Posterior half frontal lobe	Speech arrests	Lower half pre- and post-central cortex
Perisylvian area		
Posterior part 2nd temporal g.		
Posterior half frontal lobe	Speech alterations	Area around Rolandic fissure
Perisylvian area		
Posterior half frontal lobe	Aphasic disorders	
Perisylvian area		(rare)
Posterior part 2nd temporal g.		
Anterior part temporal lobe (rare)		
Parieto-temporo-occipital junction (rare)		
Temporo-parietal area	Verbal memory disturbances	

thus been mapped is responsive to electrical stimulation. On the contrary, sites where the electric current affects verbal behaviour are intermingled with sites at which this is not the case. There are also sites where electrostimulation is inconsistently effective.

Moreover, large interindividual differences have been observed in the distribution, within the area, of the sites where electrostimulation has an effect on language. Only one small zone has been discovered where the current consistently and in nearly all patients tested interferes with language. This zone occupies a small portion of the third frontal convolution just in front of the left motor strip.

Reliability of Cortical Electrostimulation

Interesting as they are, the results of electric stimulation do not enable one to predict confidently the outcome of cortical excision. The functional impairment observed during electrostimulation may differ from the functional disturbance caused by neurosurgical ablation. Indeed, the current applied to a certain area may interfere with a given function while removal of that area does not. For instance, Penfield and Welch (1951)[30] observed that electrostimulation of the mouth area in the lower sensorimotor strip could make it impossible for the patient to speak, whilst excision of this area did not greatly affect the ability to speak. Penfield and Roberts (1959, p. 129)[29] reported that of 15 patients who had shown speech arrests during electrical stimulation of a given area 10 had no aphasia after resection of that area. And Ojemann (1979)[22] described a patient who underwent left anterior temporal lobectomy. He had no postoperative aphasia although the excised region included sites at which stimulation had elicited naming errors part of the time.

Conversely, patients may be aphasic following surgery, even though pre-operative electrical stimulation did not interfere with their speech production. Penfield and Roberts (1959)[29] mentioned 11 such patients in a group of 65. And Ojemann (1979)[22] had a patient with significant aphasia following left anterior temporal lobectomy although pre-operative electrical stimulation of the area to be excised had not disturbed speech production.

Electrostimulation, then, may fail to induce verbal disturbances whilst excision of the corresponding zone results in significant language deficits. "The surgeon must be aware of this possibility", Penfield and Roberts warned (1959)[29].

How can this lack of coincidence between the results of electrical stimulation of the cortex and the effects of excision be explained?

That resection should be more detrimental to the patient's verbal performances than electrical stimulation is not difficult to understand. Removal of a continuous stretch of cortex together with some of the underlying white matter can be expected to impair the individual more than the application of a weak current to a circumscribed locus. Moreover, during electrical stimulation the patient engages in one or possibly two different verbal tasks, such as counting aloud or naming objects on confrontation. Such simple tests cannot be assumed to sample the whole of the verbal functions. Accordingly, the excision may impair linguistic skills which were not assessed during electrical stimulation.

The reverse situation is less easy to explain. Why does electrical excitation of a cortical site sometimes interfere with verbal activity while removal of an area including this site does not affect language? Penfield and Welch (1951)[30] attempted to answer this question. They suggested that electrical stimulation of a small group of neurons may irradiate, through these neurons' projections, to more distant associated circuits and perturb the performance of these circuits. Such irradiation does not take place when the neurons are removed.

In fact, the way electrostimulation interferes with verbal behaviour is still poorly understood. In particular, it is not clear why, when a particular site is stimulated on two different occasions, it may disturb language at one time and leave it unaffected the other time. As the stimulating probe is usually applied by hand, there may be slight variations in the strength with which it touches the cortex and this may conceivably have an influence on the response.

The variability observed in stimulation and stimulation effects casts some doubt on the significance of the results of cortical stimulation in bilingual individuals. If, as in a case described by Ojemann and Whitaker (1978)[27], the current, when applied at a particular frontal site, disturbs language A 3 times out of 5 and language B 1 time out of 5, is one entitled to consider that language A is more strongly represented at this site than language B? Can one really use this type of evidence to argue that in polyglots the different languages do not have identical cortical localizations (Rapport et al. 1983)[31]? It would seem that cortical electrostimulation is too crude a technique to make such subtle distinctions possible. Apart from a gross mapping of cortical areas likely to be involved in language processing, it does not allow for reliable conclusions about the cerebral mechanisms of language.

2. Subcortical Stimulation

In subcortical stimulation, a monopolar or bipolar electrode mounted on a needle or a shaft is introduced via a burr hole in the skull and pushed down to some predetermined target. At times there are several ring electrodes extending along the shaft.

Like cortical stimulation, subcortical stimulation in conscious patients may have both excitatory and inhibitory effects on speech. It may also alter speech delivery and impair linguistic competence.

Involuntary Utterances

Subcortical stimulation may cause a patient to utter words. Schaltenbrand (1965, 1975)[34,35] reported that repetitive excitation of various parts of the thalamus with fairly strong currents could elicit phrases such as "Thank you" or "Now one goes home". These unintentional utterances were often accompanied by involuntary movements of the eyes or extremities.

If stimulated several times in a row, some patients *always produced the same utterance*, while others changed utterances at every new stimulation.

On occasion the stimulation elicited words or syllables which were repeated several times. In response to a first stimulation a patient said: "Left is at my side". He reacted to the second stimulation with "Professor, I know exactly what people are talking about me". The third time, however, he stammered: "The, the, the, the".

After stimulation the patients as a rule could not remember the words which they had compulsively uttered.

Involuntary verbal reactions were observed during excitation of the left as well as of the right thalamus. They were more frequent, however, when stimulation occurred on the left.

Ojemann (1975) described a woman suffering from Parkinsonism who when initially stimulated said "That's goofy". The second, third, and fourth stimulation elicited "Twinky", even though, just before the current was applied for the fourth time, the patient had been urged to keep silent. The fifth stimulation occurred while the patient was actively counting. When the current was applied, she stopped counting, said "Twinky" and then resumed counting. On the seventh stimulation she involuntarily said "You just made the shuck go", and on the eighth stimulation, "Shucks once and a while".

Such verbal ejaculations are somewhat reminiscent of the uncontrollable utterances of some patients with extrapyramidal diseases and of the coprolalias of patients with Gilles de la Tourette's syndrome.

When it has an excitatory effect on verbal behaviour, subcortical stimulation, then, tends to elicit more complex utterances than cortical stimulation.

However, Schaltenbrand (1965, 1975)[34,35] reported that at times yells, clicks, or some other nonverbal sounds were produced instead of words. Under the influence of the electric current applied to the thalamus, some patients coughed, swallowed, or licked their lips. Similar observations were made by Van Buren (1963)[40] during stimulation in the vicinity of the head of the caudate nucleus.

Speech Arrests

Arrest of both verbal and motor activity was occasionally observed by Ojemann et al. (1968)[24] during stimulation of the parietal white matter in the right as well as in the left hemisphere. Stimulation of this subcortical area could also cause unpleasant sensations or lassitude and disinterest, which then interfered with naming activities.

Schaltenbrand (1965)[34] reported speech arrests following repetitive electrical stimulation of the radiations of the corpus callosum, presumably in either hemisphere.

Van Buren (1963)[40] repeatedly noted speech arrests during electrostimulation in the vicinity of the head of the caudate nucleus in the right as well as in the left hemisphere. When asked afterwards why they had stopped talking, the patients tended to give unlikely answers or inconsequent excuses which testified to some transient poststimulation confusion. Van Buren (1966) pointed out that the speech arrests could be accompanied by slow contralateral deviation of the head and eyes.

Speech Alterations

In one left-handed patient Ojemann et al. (1968)[24] noted that stimulation of the left thalamus consistently caused stutter-like repetition of the first part of words produced in a naming-on-confrontation test. The same type of repetition was observed by Ojemann (1976)[21] in two right-handers. For example, in response to a picture of a telephone the patient would say "This is a tele-tele-tele" (the current was then turned off) "a telephone".

Several investigators, including Guiot et al. (1961)[10], noted that subcortical electrostimulation could cause an involuntary acceleration of speech delivery. The patients generally were aware of their tachyphemia but could not suppress it. One of the patients of Guiot et al. (1961)[10], when asked why he had spoken precipitously when stimulation was applied, said: "There was something in me which forced me to hurry".

The acceleration in delivery may outlast the stimulation by a few minutes. At other times, it ends, during stimulation, in an inaudible whisper. When the latter occurs, accelerated and audible delivery may be resumed after a few seconds.

Aphasic Disturbances

A tendency to misname common objects or to fail to name them although the ability to speak was retained (= anomia), could be observed by Ojemann et al. (1968)[24] during stimulation of the left thalamus, particularly of the left pulvinar, in right-handed patients. In one left-hander, stimulation of the right pulvinar also resulted in occasional misnaming or anomia.

Anomia could also be brought on by stimulation

Table 2. *Sub-Cortical Stimulation*

Sites in the left hemisphere	Verbal behaviours	Sites in the right hemisphere
Thalamus	Involuntary utterances	Thalamus
Parietal white matter	Speech arrests	Parietal white matter
Radiations corpus callosum		Radiations corpus callosum
Caudate nucleus		Caudate nucleus
Thalamus	Speech alterations	
Thalamus	Aphasic disturbances	Thalamus (rare)
Parietal white matter		Parietal white matter

of the parietal white matter in the left as well as in the right hemisphere of right-handers. At times, electric stimulation at these various sites resulted in an increase of the response latency. The response, however, was adequate.

Ojemann (1975)[20] also mentioned anomia after left thalamic stimulation and after stimulation of the right internal capsule.

Short Term Verbal Memory

Ojemann et al. (1971)[25] found that subcortical (and more specifically, thalamic) stimulation on the left during naming tended to decrease the number of errors when the patients had to recall the name they had given to a particular object a little earlier. On the contrary, stimulation at the time of recall tended to increase the number of errors. In other words, stimulation during the verbal response to be remembered enhanced the memory of it, whilst stimulation during recollection had a negative influence on mnesic performance.

3. *Cortical vs. Sub-Cortical Stimulation*

Sub-cortical electrostimulation, then, may have various effects on verbal behaviour. Some of these effects resemble those observed during cortical stimulation, others are different. As is the case with stimulation of the cortex, effects are more frequent when the current is applied to the left, than when it is applied to the right, hemisphere.

Resective Surgery

Ablation of cerebral tissue performed with a view to alleviating otherwise intractable epilepsy is generally limited to one lobe. Resection involving the temporal lobe usually includes the temporal tip and may extend back far enough to encompass the transverse gyri of Heschel. On the mesial aspect, the removal ordinarily includes the amygdala and may or may not encroach upon the hippocampus. As a rule the neurosurgeon avoids invading the zones in which electrostimulation has interfered with verbal behaviour.

Frontal resection ordinarily includes the frontal pole and, on the mesial surface, may extend to parts of the cingulate and subcallosal gyri. Broca's area, on the other hand, is most of the time spared.

In the parietal lobe, excisions are more variable in locus and extent. They tend to avoid areas when electrostimulation has interfered with verbal behaviour.

Naming-on-Confrontation

Wilkins and Moscovitch (1978)[43] found that a group of patients having undergone left anterior temporal lobectomy for intractable epilepsy scored significantly below norm on a naming-on-confrontation test. The subjects had been operated upon 1 to 21 years before testing. It is not known whether they had some degree of anomia pre-operatively.

Short Term Verbal Memory

Milner (1962, 1967)[17,18] studied short term verbal memory in epileptic patients before and after left anterior temporal resection. She examined both delayed verbal associative learning and delayed story recall. The patients had to remember pairs of words that had been read out to them some time previously or to recall as many details as possible from a story they had been told a little earlier. A written version of these tests was also administered.

Milner found that compared to patients with an epileptogenic focus in the right temporal lobe, patients with a focus on the left had reduced short term verbal memory pre-operatively. This reduction increased after surgical resection, especially when the verbal material to be remembered was presented auditorily. This postoperative impairment did not significantly improve over the years. In some cases it was associated with some degree of aphasia immediately after surgery. The aphasia soon cleared up whilst the verbal memory deficit remained. Patients who were taking courses at school or university complained that they had more difficulty than formerly in apprehending the material presented. One year after lobectomy, one of these patients, an intelligent young man, explained that when trying to learn new words, he could hardly remember more than one out of five after three of four days.

The mean I.Q.'s of the patients with left and of the patients with right temporal lesions were quite similar.

Therefore, the short term verbal memory impairment of the patients with left temporal resection could not be viewed as the consequence of a general intellectual deterioration. Accordingly, Milner concluded that "the evidence for a residual impairment of verbal memory several years after temporal lobectomy is compelling and contrasts with the normal verbal recall of patients with comparable excisions in other parts of the cerebral cortex".

The significant decline in short term verbal memory observed in patients with left temporal lobectomies tended to correlate with both the lateral and medial extent of the ablation.

Milner's findings were confirmed by Ojemann and Dodrill (1985)[23] who assessed short term verbal memory in a dozen epileptic patients. The task required the patients to recall as many details as possible from a story that had just been read out to them. The subjects were tested before temporal lobe resection, at one month post-op. and at one year post-op.

One month after operation 8 out of 13 patients evidenced a reduction of short term verbal memory as compared with their pre-operative scores. Two patients showed no change and 3 showed an improvement.

One year after operation the deficit was found to have increased further in five of the eight cases which had shown a reduction of short term verbal memory at one month follow-up. None of these five patients was seizure-free post-operatively. The verbal memory decline correlated with the lateral but not with the mesial extent of the resection.

Falconer (in Darley and Millikan, 1967, p. 139)[7] remarked that in his experience the impairment of short term verbal memory observed in patients with left temporal lobectomies tends to decrease with the passing of time, at least in subjects who are seizure-free after operation. He quoted the case of a bilingual adult who several years after operation managed to acquire a third language.

Milner (1962, 1967)[17,18] also studied the effect of left frontal lobectomy on verbal recall. She found no evidence of a reduction of short term verbal memory.

Verbal Fluency

Verbal fluency is the ability to generate lists of words beginning with a given letter or belonging to a semantic category (such as fruit or clothing) specified by the examiner.

Martin *et al.* (1990)[16] studied word fluency in patients with unilateral temporal lobe epilepsy both before and after anterior temporal lobectomy. Regardless of the side of the epileptogenic focus, the scores of the patients were significantly lower than those of healthy controls, with patients with left temporal lobe epilepsy more impaired than patients with right temporal lobe epilepsy. This was true both before and after operation.

Post-operative testing took place one week after anterior temporal lobectomy. Mean results indicated poorer performances after operation in both groups of patients.

Milner (1962, 1967)[17,18] compared the verbal fluency test scores of patients who had undergone left frontal, right frontal, or left temporal lobectomies. She found that the scores of the left frontal group were more depressed than those of the other two groups. Moreover, she noted that patients who had undergone left frontal lobectomy tended to lack spontaneous speech.

Thus, temporal lobectomy for the control of intractable epilepsy generally increases the pre-operative deficit in short term verbal memory and in verbal fluency. With the passing of time, the impairment may return to its pre-operative level, especially in patients who are seizure-free after operation.

Frontal lobectomy, on the other hand, does not seem to affect short term verbal memory but tends to deplete verbal fluency scores more severely than temporal lobectomy, especially if it is performed on the left side.

These, however, are all group observations. There must be individual exceptions. At times temporal lobectomy interferes little, if at all, with language processing. For instance, one of Wilkins and Moscovitch's left lobectomy patients (1978) had a Wechsler verbal I.Q. of 138. And, as was mentioned above, one of Falconer's bilingual patients was able to acquire a third language after operation. It is possible that such favorable conditions never occur shortly after operation and occur only in seizure-free patients.

Stereotaxic Surgery

In an effort to alleviate involuntary movements, tremor, or intractable pain, neurosurgeons may place a lesion in the thalamus, the internal capsule or the globus pallidus. The surgical target in the case of thalamotomy is often the ventrolateral nucleus. However, at times lesions are made in the pulvinar.

The operation may be unilateral, or on the contrary be a staged bilateral procedure. A stylus is introduced via a burr hole in the skull and pushed down to the desired target. The lesion is made by thermo-electric coagulation, freezing (cryogenic technique) or injection of alcohol. This last procedure is now almost obsolete.

Stereotaxic surgery on subcortical structures not infrequently entails temporary or lasting neurolinguistic deficits.

Mutism

Mutism of some two weeks' duration was observed by Botez and Barbeau (1971)[4] after left thalamotomy in two patients who had had right thalamotomy a few years before. After the period of mutism, anomia was in evidence for 6–9 months. The patients' delivery was rendered hesitant by the word finding difficulties.

Gross and Kuhner (1969)[9] noted that thalamotomy could occasionally be followed by akinetic mutism.

Voice

Gros and Kuhner (1969)[9] observed postoperative aphonia in a number of cases, especially after bilateral thalamotomy. They did not report whether this condition improved over time. They also noted that in a few patients who had pre-operative aphonia, voice production was improved after surgery. A similar observation was made by Krayenbühl *et al.* (1963)[13].

In a group of 37 parkinsonian patients who had had a left stereotaxic operation, Allan *et al.* (1966)[1] found 25 (67%) whose voice volume had decreased after the procedure. The same was observed in 16 (36%) of 44 patients who had had a right-sided operation. Of the 53 patients who had had bilateral operations 30 (56%) showed decreased voice volume post-operatively.

However, the effect of stereotaxic surgery on vocal volume may also be positive. Of 74 patients who had hypophonia before operation, 26 (35%) had improved vocal volume postoperatively.

At times, the operation leaves vocal volume unchanged. This was observed in 21 of 60 patients who before operation had normal or near normal vocal intensity.

Bell (1968)[3] noted that after operation voice volume could be reduced to the point of inaudibility. Reduction of vocal intensity was more frequent after bilateral than after unilateral thalamotomy. It tended to improve over the first few weeks after operation.

Stereotaxic procedures, then, may entail an impairment or, on the contrary, an improvement, of voice production. Decrease in vocal volume tends to be more frequent than increase, especially after left-sided operation. Apparently, patients who have preoperative reduced vocal volume tend to improve afterwards, whereas deterioration occurs primarily in patients with previously normal voice production.

Articulation

In a group of 53 patients who had undergone bilateral thalamotomy or pallidotomy on one side and thalamotomy on the other, Krayenbühl et al. (1961)[12] found 24 cases with deterioration, and 13 cases with improvement, of articulation. Dysarthria could be observed even though operation had resulted in a marked reduction of rigidity.

Allan et al. (1966)[1] and Hermann et al. (1966)[11] confirmed that articulation could deteriorate after stereotaxic surgery, particularly when the lesion was made on the left side or was bilateral. Fifty-four per cent of their parkinsonian patients who had had left-sided operation, 36% of their patients who had had right-sided operation, and 66% of their patients who had had a bilateral procedure, showed a postoperative deterioration of articulation. However, a few patients who had pre-operative dysarthria spoke more clearly after operation.

Krayenbühl et al. (1963)[13] felt that if unilateral operation is followed by some dysarthria, this articulatory disorder is likely to increase if the patient undergoes stereotaxy on the other side. In a similar vein, Selby (1967)[36] warned that in patients with pre-operative slurring of speech the risk of having pronounced dysarthria after a bilateral operation is really great.

Bell (1968)[3] noted that following surgery a few patients had difficulty in initiating speech. The starting mechanism of speech appeared impaired.

In a few cases, Samra et al. (1969)[33] observed a postoperative change in rate of delivery. There was either tachyphemia or bradyphemia.

Examining parkinsonian patients three to six years after unilateral stereotaxy, Krayenbühl et al. (1963)[13] found that about one third of them had dysarthria or hypophonia. It was not clear, however, whether this was a direct consequence of the operation or of the degenerative disease itself or of both combined.

Stereotaxic surgery, then, may affect articulation negatively, particularly if it is performed on the left-side or is bilateral. However, occasionally it may result in an improvement of articulation. Postoperative dysarthria may be a lasting condition.

Language

Transient aphasia was observed by Allan et al. (1966)[1] and by Hermann et al. (1966)[11] in a few right-handed patients after a left-sided or bilateral stereotaxic operation. Svennilson et al. (1960)[39] found that following left unilateral stereotaxy transitory aphasia was more frequent in patients with pre-operative cerebral atrophy (as measured by ventricular dilation) than in patients without such atrophy.

Using Schuell's Short Test for Aphasia, Darley et al. (1975)[7] found that in a group of 101 patients who had undergone thalamotomy, 20 showed some deterioration of their linguistic competence shortly after operation. Of 22 patients who had undergone pallidectomy alone or pallidectomy followed by thalamotomy 8 evidenced a similar deterioration.

Language change occurred about twice as often in cases of left thalamotomy as in cases of right thalamotomy. Moreover, patients who underwent single unilateral thalamotomy suffered a much lower incidence of language deterioration than those with multiple unilateral thalamotomies.

In Botez and Barbeau's opinion (1971)[4] thalamotomy never results in lasting receptive language disorders. In other words, it never impairs verbal comprehension permanently. As a matter of fact, in a group of 118 parkinsonian patients who had undergone stereotactic thalamotomy, Allan et al. (1966)[1] found sensory aphasia only occasionally. The deficit proved to be temporary in all cases. It cleared up entirely within a few weeks.

Yet Vilkki and Laitinen (1974)[42] noted that 6 to 18 months after unilateral thalamotomy, patients operated upon on the left side tended to have longer reaction times to verbal orders than patients operated upon on the right side.

Krayenbühl et al. (1965)[14] compared the pre- and post-operative scores on a short term verbal memory test of patients having undergone left-sided or right-sided stereotaxic operation. They found that immediately after operation the scores of patients with left-sided lesions showed a statistically significant decrease. This was not observed in the group of patients with right-sided lesions. The test required the patients to memorize a series of words read out by the examiner.

Ojemann et al. (1971)[25] also observed some reduction of short term verbal memory after left but not after right thalamotomy. This reduction was apparent when the delay period between the naming of an object by the patient and his recall of his own naming exceeded 20 seconds.

Furthermore, there was some correlation between the reduction in short-term verbal memory and the patient's reactions to pre-operative electrostimulation of the thalamus. When electrostimulation during naming improved subsequent recall whilst electro-stimulation during recall significantly worsened the patient's memory performance, there tended to be a post-operative deficit in short term verbal memory.

Almgren *et al.* (1972)[2] compared right-handed patients with left, and right-handed patients with right, ventrolateral thalamotomy on the Stroop Colour Test and on a memory test of word pairs. In the first part of the Stroop Colour Test, the subjects had to tell the printing colour of a number of printed words which were no colour-names. In the second part they had to tell the printing colour of a number of colour names, with the printing colour and the name of the colour never corresponding (e.g. the word "blue" was printed in yellow, green or red ink, but never in blue ink).

In the memory test of word pairs used by Almgren *et al.*, the subjects were asked to memorize word pairs (e.g. sun-shadow, chair-pillow...) which the experimenter read aloud from a printed list also available to the subjects. After ten word pairs had been read, the list was removed and the experimenter said the first word of each pair in an order different from that of the list. The subjects had to respond with the second word. Three lists of ten word pairs each were used successively.

Pre-operatively, there was no significant difference between the two groups of patients on these two tests. Shortly after operation patients with left thalamotomy proved as a group, significantly impaired on the verbal memory test and on the second part on the Stroop Colour Test, while patients with right thalamotomy tended to perform better than before operation.

When retested several months later, the group of patients with left thalamotomy proved less impaired than immediately after operation. In fact, overall performance nearly equalled pre-operative results. The performance of the group of patients with right thalamotomy was roughly the same as immediately after operation. The two groups still differed in one respect viz. the scores on the second part of the Stroop Colour Test.

Comparing pre-operative verbal I.Q.'s with post-operative verbal I.Q.'s measured immediately after operation and again 12 to 31 months after operation, Shapiro *et al.* (1973)[37] found a greater mean decline in the group of parkinsonian patients who had undergone left unilateral thalamotomy than in the group of parkinsonian patients who had had right unilateral thalamotomy. At the individual level, the drop in scores tended to increase with the patient's age.

Riklan *et al.* (1969)[32] compared the scores on a verbal fluency test of parkinsonian patients before and after stereotaxy. Significant score changes occurred imme-diately postoperatively only in the case of left hemisphere operations. After several months the patients who had undergone left-side operation were found to have returned essentially to their pre-operative level.

A test in which the patients had to detect an odd word in a group of three yielded similar results. In addition, it was found that patients with bilateral operation scored essentially like patients with left unilateral operation.

Several months after operation Ojemann *et al.* (1971)[25] noted a slight decrease of the scores on an object-naming test after right or left thalamotomy in right-handed parkinsonian patients. The increase in error rate was larger after a left-sided lesion.

Graphomotricity

Selective thalamotomy was performed in a limited number of patients with a view to alleviating primary writing tremor. The latter is a tremor which appears only when the patient attempts to write.

In a patient whose writing tremor was so severe that he could not write a single word legibly, Siegfried *et al.* (1969)[38] performed a series of three electrocoagulations in the ventrolateral nucleus of the left thalamus. After each coagulation, graphomotricity improved. After the third one, it was essentially normal. Three months after operation script was still quite adequate.

In three cases of primary writing tremor, Ohye *et al.* (1982)[19] performed electrocoagulation centred on the nucleus ventralis intermedius. In one of these cases thalamotomy had to be repeated twice before writing tremor could be completely eliminated. In the other two cases, one operation sufficed to produce a cure.

Improvement of writing was also noted by Hermann *et al.* (1966)[11] in a left-handed patient after right-sided stereotaxy. The operation reduced tremor and rigidity, which in turn resulted in better penmanship.

In patients who had undergone bilateral operation for the treatment of Parkinsonism, Krayenbühl *et al.* (1961)[12] occasionally noted a reduction of both dysarthria and micrographia.

Stereotaxy, then, may improve graphomotricity, whether writing movements are selectively disturbed by tremor or are impaired by an overall rigidity.

It thus appears that stereotaxic surgery may entail changes in language, speech, and writing.

Some degree of aphasia may be observed immediately after operation. It is more frequent after left-sided than after right-sided lesions. Usually, it is transient. However, word-finding difficulties with resultant hesitancy of speech may last longer. There may also be some durable loss of metalinguistic agility as measured by such tests as the Stroop Colour Test.

Occasionally transient mutism is observed immediately after operation.

It is still a matter of debate whether aphasia consequent upon stereotaxic surgery is due to the probe tract through the cortex and subjacent structures, to the perilesional œdema, to haemorrhage or infarct, or to the surgical sub-cortical lesion proper.

Speech also may be altered following stereotaxy. There may be postoperative slurring of speech and even frank dysarthria, especially after left-sided or bilateral operation. This postoperative dysarthria may be a lasting condition.

At times, however, pre-operative dysarthria appears improved following stereotaxy.

The same holds true in respect of voice production. After surgery vocal volume may be reduced. But in patients who had pre-operative hypo- or aphonia, the surgical procedure may result in improved voice production. When stereotaxy is followed by a decrease in vocal volume, this sequela may be transient or durable.

When graphomotricity is disturbed by tremor or rigidity, stereotaxy, by eliminating the trembling or reducing the hypertonia, may improve the quality of penmanship.

Conclusions

Medically intractable focal epilepsy can often be relieved by resection of the epileptogenic cortical area. Such resection, especially when it is performed on the left hemisphere, may result in lasting and incapacitating language impairments. Neurosurgeons, therefore, are careful to avoid resecting areas whose ablation could compromise the patient's linguistic functioning.

To some extent, the limits of cortical regions that should be spared vary from patient to patient. Accordingly, the surgeon usually attempts to delineate the sites he should avoid injuring in any individual patient who is to be operated upon. Most of the time electrostimulation is used to this end.

Electrostimulation of the cortex may have both excitatory and inhibitory effects on verbal behaviour. At some places, the current elicits involuntary vocalizations, at other places it disturbs linguistic processing by the brain or impedes verbal expression.

Electrostimulation is also used before stereotaxic operations in an effort to anticipate the results and

possible consequences of iatrogenic destruction of some sub-cortical sites. The current applied to various sub-cortical structures may equally interfere with voluntary verbal behaviour or elicit involuntary verbal reactions.

Resections which avoid sites where interference with language or speech has been observed during electric stimulation may nevertheless result in some neurolinguistic impairment. Left anterior temporal lobectomy may entail a deficit in verbal recall which may persist for several years, and left anterior frontal lobectomy may entail a decline in verbal fluency and a reduction of spontaneous speech.

These negative consequences of partial lobectomy should probably, in each individual case, be weighed against the possible gain in quality of life resulting from the alleviation of epilepsy.

Stereotaxic operations performed on the left side may entail transient aphasia and even, occasionally, transient mutism. After left-sided or bilateral procedures, there may also be a reduction of metalinguistic abilities, which may or may not improve after some time.

Stereotaxic surgery may further bring about a lasting deterioration of articulation and a lasting reduction of voice volume, particularly after bilateral operation. When contemplating stereotaxy, these hazards should not be ignored, as the iatrogenic deficit in speech and voice production may largely outweigh the motor benefits of the surgical procedure. On the other hand, it should be remembered that operation may occasionally result in an improvement of speech or voice. Unfortunately, it does not seem possible, at the present time, to predict in any individual case whether operation will have a positive or a negative effect, or no effect at all, on speaking and voicing.

References

1. Allan C, Turner J, Gadea-Ciria M (1966) Investigations into speech disturbances following stereotaxic surgery for parkinsonism. Br J Disord Commun 1: 55–59
2. Almgren P, Andersson A, Kullberg G (1972) Long-term effects on verbally expressed cognition following left and right ventrolateral thalamotomy. Confina Neurologica 34: 162–168
3. Bell D (1968) Speech functions of the thalamus inferred from the effects of thalamotomy. Brain 91: 619–638
4. Botez M, Barbeau A (1971) Role of subcortical structures and particularly the thalamus, in the mechanisms of speech and language. Int J Neurol 8: 300–320
5. Brickner R (1940) A human critical area producing repetitive phenomena when stimulated. J Neurophysiol 3: 128–130
6. Darley F, Brown J, Swenson W (1975) Language changes after neurosurgery for Parkinsonism. Brain and Language 2: 65–69

7. Darley F, Millikan C (1967) Brain mechanisms underlying speech and language. Grune and Stratton, New York
8. Fedio P, Van Buren J (1974) Memory deficits during electrical stimulation of the speech cortex in conscious man. Brain and Language 1: 29–42
9. Gros C, Kuhner A (1969) Thalamotomie bilatérale. La Journée du Thalamus. Paris, Drop, pp 105–108
10. Guiot G, Hertzog E, Rondot P, Molina P (1961) Arrest or acceleration of speech evoked by thalamic stimulation in the course of stereotaxic procedures for parkinsonism. Brain 84: 363–369
11. Hermann K, Turner J, Gillingham F, Gaze R (1966) The effects of destructive lesions and stimulation of the basal ganglia on speech mechanisms. Confina Neurologica 27: 197–207
12. Krayenbühl H, Wyss O, Yaşargil M (1961) Bilateral thalamotomy and pallidotomy as treatment for bilateral Parkinsonism. J Neurosurg 18: 429–444
13. Krayenbühl H, Siegfried J, Yaşargil M (1963) Resultats tardifs des opérations stéréotaxiques dans le traitement de la maladie du Parkinson. Rev Neurol (Paris) 108: 485–494
14. Krayenbühl H, Siegfried J, Kohenof M, Yaşargil M (1965) Is there a dominant thalamus? Confina neurologica 26: 246–249
15. Lesser R, Lueders H, Dinner D, Hahn J, Cohen L (1984) The location of speech and writing functions in the frontal language area. Brain 107: 275–291
16. Martin R, Loring D, Meador K, Lee G (1990) The effects of lateralized temporal lobe dysfunction on formal and semantic word fluency. Neuropsychologia 28: 823–829
17. Milner B (1962) Laterality effects in audition. In: Mountcastle V (ed) Interhemispheric relations and cerebral dominance. Baltimore, The Johns Hopkins Press, pp 177–195
18. Milner B (1967) Brain mechanisms suggested by studies of temporal lobes. In: Darley F, Millikan C (eds) Brain mechanisms underlying speech and language. Grune & Stratton, New York, pp 122–132
19. Ohye C, Miyazaki M, Hirai T, Shibazaki T, Nakajima H, Nagaseki Y (1982) Primary writing tremor treated by stereotactic selective thalamotomy. J Neurol Neurosurg Psychiat 45: 988–997
20. Ojemann G (1975) Language and the thalamus: Object naming and recall during and after thalamic stimulation. Brain and Language 2: 101–120
21. Ojemann G (1976) Subcortical language mechanisms. In: Whitaker H (ed) Studies in neurolinguistics, Vol 1. Academic Press, New York, pp 103–138
22. Ojemann G (1979) Individual variability in cortical localization of language. J Neurosurg 50: 164–169
23. Ojemann G, Dodrill C (1985) Verbal memory deficits after left temporal lobectomy for epilepsy. J Neurosurg 62: 101–107
24. Ojemann G, Fedio P, Van Buren J (1968) Anomia from pulvinar and subcortical parietal stimulation. Brain 91: 99–116
25. Ojemann G, Hoyenga K, Ward A (1971) Prediction of short-term verbal memory disturbance after ventrolateral thalamotomy. J Neurosurg 35: 203–210
26. Ojemann G, Ojemann J, Lettich E, Berger M (1989) Cortical language localization in left, dominant hemisphere. J Neurosurg 71: 316–326
27. Ojemann G, Whitaker H (1978) The bilingual brain. Arch Neurol 35: 409–412
28. Penfield W (1938) The cerebral cortex in man. I. The cerebral cortex and consciousness. Arch Neurol Psychiat 40: 417–442
29. Penfield W, Roberts L (1959) Speech and brain mechanisms. Princeton University Press, Princeton (NJ)
30. Penfield W, Welch K (1951) The supplementary motor area of the cerebral cortex. Arch Neurol Psychiat 66: 289–317
31. Rapport R, Tan C, Whitaker H (1983) Language function and dysfunction among Chinese- and English-speaking polyglots: Cortical stimulation, Wada testing and clinical studies. Brain and Language 18: 342–366
32. Riklan M, Levita E, Zimmerman J, Cooper I (1969) Thalamic correlates of language and speech. J Neurol Sci 8: 307–328
33. Samra K, Riklan M, Levita E, Zimmerman J, Waltz J, Bergmann L, Cooper I (1969) Language and speech correlates of anatomically verified lesions in thalamic surgery for parkinsonism. J Speech Hear Res 12: 510–540
34. Schaltenbrand G (1965) The effects of stereotactic electrical stimulation in the depth of the brain. Brain 88: 835–840
35. Schaltenbrand G (1975) The effects on speech and language of stereotactical stimulation in thalamus and corpus callosum. Brain and Language 2: 70–77
36. Selby G (1967) Stereotactic surgery for the relief of Parkinson's disease. Part II: Analysis of the results in a series of 303 patients (413 operations). J Neurol Sci 5: 343–375
37. Shapiro D, Sadowsky D, Henderson W, Van Buren J (1973) An assessment of cognitive function in post-thalamotomy Parkinson patients. Confina Neurologica 35: 144–166
38. Siegfried J, Crowell R, Perret E (1969) Cure of tremulous writer's cramp by stereotaxic thalamotomy. J Neurosurg 30: 182–185
39. Svennilson E, Torvik A, Lower R, Kesell L (1960) Treatment of parkinsonism by stereotactic thermolesions in the pallidal region. Acta Psychiat Neurol Scand 35: 358–377
40. Van Buren J (1963) Confusion and disturbance of speech from stimulation in vicinity of the head of the caudate nucleus. J Neurosurg 20: 148–157
41. Van Buren J, Fedio P, Frederick G (1978) Mechanism and localization of speech in the parietotemporal cortex. Neurosurgery 2: 233–239
42. Vilkki J, Laitinen L (1974) Differential effects of left and right ventrolateral thalamotomy on receptive and expressive verbal performances and face-matching. Neuropsychologia 12: 11–19
42. Whitaker H, Ojemann G (1977) Graded localisation of naming from electrical stimulation mapping of left cerebral cortex. Nature 270: 50–51
43. Wilkins A, Moscovitch M (1978) Selective impairment of semantic memory after temporal lobectomy. Neuropsychologia 16: 73–79

Correspondence: Y. Lebrun, Neurolinguistics, School of Medicine, Vrije Universiteit, Brussel, Laarbeeklaan 103, 1090 Brussels, Belgium.

Acta Neurochirurgica (1993) [Suppl] 56: 52–58

Clinical Forms of Aphasia

A. Kertesz

Department of Clinical Neurological Sciences, St. Joseph's Hospital, London, Ont., Canada

Summary

A survey is given on the history of knowledge of aphasia and on the necessity and possibilities of classification of aphasic disability. Also the association of clinical syndromes of aphasia with particular damage to the brain is outlined.

For Wernicke's aphasia (fluent aphasia with comprehension deficit) a superior posterior temporal lesion is obligatory. The persistent jargon aphasia is associated with a lesion of the supramarginal gyrus. Broca's aphasia is seen with posterior inferior frontal leisons, but additional central and subcortical components are involved in persisting deficit. The lesions producing transcortical motor aphasia involve the supplementary speech area of Penfield. Transcortical sensory aphasia is related to lesions that overlap the watershed area between the middle cerebral and the posterior cerebral arteries.

Keywords: Aphasia; syndromes; classification; morphological correlation.

Inroduction

It is a pleasure to be invited to give a talk at this high level academic gathering, and it is a particular pleasure for me, personally, to be a guest because I spent the first 20 years of my life here in Budapest. Last night, I walked out on the fisherman's bastion and looked on the city in its floodlit beauty, and I said to myself there isn't really any other city like this in the world. So I think special thanks are due to Dr. Pasztor and Dr. Vajda and their particularly able team, putting up a conference at this particular venue, and in the name of invited guests, I would like to express my appreciation.

I am going to talk about the classification, assessment and some of the biological and anatomical features of aphasic disability. We should first ask the question whether we need any classification of aphasia. Do we need to talk about clinical forms of aphasia, or is this *just one of these* academic exercises nurologists like to get involved in? Some clinicians will say, when the speech is impaired, it is aphasia, and that is all there is to it. There are little differences, certain aspects are a little bit more severe, a little less severe, but is there really any point arguing about what kind of aphasia it is? I hope to show that yes, classification is useful.

The other related issue I would like to discuss is, that if there are clinical forms of aphasia, are they associated with particular injury to the brain, in other words, is there such a thing as localization for certain aphasic syndromes? I emphasize "syndromes" and not symptoms, because I do not believe that you can localize symptoms to parts of the brain. For instance, I do not believe that you can localize the function of comprehension much more than you can localize the function of sisterly love, or patriotism. I believe, and the evidence from physiological methods is very convincing, that the brain is activated for complex functions in a widely spread fashion. Anybody who has seen the pictures of glucose metabolism of people reading for instance, has a pretty clear idea that not only the occipital lobe, but Wernicke's area, Broca's area, supplementary motor area, and furthermore, the other hemisphere are also activated. Even when a single word, for instance, the word "orange" is flashed on a screen or is spoken to you, not only the auditory images of the phonetic components o-r-a-n-dzs are evoked, but also associations immediately to color, smell, a trip to Florida, the last advertisement you have seen on television for orange juice, etc., etc. Relevant associations that are important for you contextually, activate much of the brain at a particular time and might be quite different from another person, or for you another time, in another context. Instead of discussing language function and brain activation further, we are going to explore the clinical forms of aphasia that have certain heuristic value for the neurological clinician and I will emphasize those particular forms that are important from the point of view of a neurosurgical practice.

The first great classification debate was going on at the end of last century. Pierre Marie (1906)[12] was very much against dividing aphasia. He said "aphasie et une" and he was not going to acknowledge any other types of aphasia. Interestingly, in 1917 he changed his mind, because at that time a great deal of neurosurgical experience with the head injured from the first world war became available. In his volume "Les Aphasies de Guerre" he said, "There is anarthria, then there is anarthria with aphasia, there is temporal aphasia, there is angular gyrus aphasia and there is global aphasia". So he ended up classifying just like everybody else, who see patients with aphasic syndromes. The question is, how *much* do we classify and what is the goal of the taxonomy? The purpose can be diagnostic, and such classifications are usually modality oriented. Classifications greatly depend on what is being tested. Are we testing comprehension? Are we testing spontaneous speech? Are we testing reading, writing, etc.? Most diagnostic aphasia tests will provide a modality oriented system. The prognostic classification considers how the aphasic syndromes evolve in time, and how the patient recovers. The therapeutic classification can be linguistic or behavioral. If the therapeutic orientation is psycholinguistic, then the patient is classified along psycholinguistic lines. Behaviorism pays attention to motivation, attention, and depression. There is also a classification which is based on neuroanatomical methods, and this explores the relationship of the speech disturbance to the lesion.

An optimal classification should be based on measurements. Scientific classification is called numerical taxonomy. The more a classification is based on measurements, the closer it comes to objective groupings that reflect reality. Classification also has to be relevant to several goals to enjoy widespread acceptance. An important principle of numerical taxonomy is that the intergroup differences have to be greater than within group differences. Classifications often violate this particular rule. Another rule is that unclassifiables should be kept to a minimum. There are systems of aphasia classification that will place only typical patients in groups and the rest are called mixed aphasics. Surprisingly, many clinicians will be satisfied with that, and some researchers will exclude them from study. For several reasons, such as therapeutic, prognostic or statistical, this is not acceptable.

In order to measure aphasic disability, one has to have an aphasia test that is reliable; it has to be applicable to a range of severity of aphasics, and it should explore all potentially disturbed modalities. It should have content validity, and the subtests should discriminate between clinical aphasia types. Many well known aphasia tests do not do this. For instance, the Porch Index of Communicative Ability (PICA, 1971)[16] does not distinguish between aphasia types. There should be graded items that sample a representative range of severity. In other words, if you only use difficult items, you might be able to differentiate between a mildly affected patient such as the Token Test does, but if you do not use easier items, you will have a floor effect, that is, many of the severely or moderately severely affected aphasics will perform equally poorly on the test. The number of items has to be numerous enough to decrease the test to test variability. There has to be a standardized scoring and administration. For instance, if the test is administered by two different persons, it has to have the same results (inter-tester reliability). It has to be practical in length; some aphasia tests are too long. It has to minimize the effect of education and intelligence. In other words, it should measure language! It has to discriminate between aphasics and others, such as the mentally retarded or patients with depression (content validity). It has to have internal consistency which is measured by the relationship of the items.

The two sine qua non items of aphasia testing are spontaneous speech and comprehension. In the absence of appropriate scoring established for these, you really cannot judge either severity or aphasia type. Repetition and naming are the other important items, and will be discussed later.

Fluency of spontaneous or conversational speech is a measure of the amount of speech output. The rate of speech is closely related to fluency. Phrase length is also related, but depends on the complexity of the phrases and grammaticality. Articulatory ability has a phonological and a prosodic component. The latter can be linguistic prosody such as asking a question or exclaiming, or emotional prosody which will tell you whether the speaker is angry or sad. The articulatory component has a well established left hemisphere mechanism, but prosodic input is claimed to be right hemispheric, especially for emotional prosody. Paraphasias are the most specific diagnostic features of the aphasic symptomatology in spontaneous or responsive speech. They are classified as phonemic (literal) or semantic (verbal). Word finding difficulty by itself is also very characteristic and important, but not necessarily diagnostic of aphasia. Finally, the information content of speech output can be scored, and it reflects the severity of aphasia.

Comprehension should be measured by several methods. For instance, if it is tested only by sentence comprehension, then you will get a very high level of comprehension measure; but if you use yes/no questions, then you are able to measure the comprehension in severe Broca's aphasics who cannot express any other way whether they know the meaning, except yes and no. Most of the time, head nodding is the most practical way of finding out even if a very mute, very severe Broca's aphasic comprehends or not. At a higher level, one can measure syntactic comprehension, whether the patient can understand grammar, and one can increase the semantic complexity of the items and vary the length of the items to be comprehended, provided care is taken not to overload short term memory (about 8 items).

Other important subtests are repetition, which is important to distinguish conduction aphasia and the transcortical aphasias. In case of conduction aphasia, it is the only subtest that is significantly affected, in contrast to the transcortical aphasias where repetition is characteristically better than some of the other language subtests. Naming is tested in all language examinations and we have developed a special naming score which takes into consideration, visual naming on confrontation, tactile naming, as well as naming phonemic and semantic cues and naming in semantic context. We also test word fluency, or producing the names of animals in one minute, and sentence completion.

We constructed an aphasia test along these lines and standardized it. The results I am presenting to you about various aphasic syndromes and their recovery are based on this aphasia test which my colleagues and I have developed at the University of Western Ontario

in London, Ontario, and published it as the Western Aphasia Battery[9,10].

The clinical typology of aphasias began with Broca (1861)[2]. I might mention that Broca was not a neurologist, but a Professor of External Surgery as they called trauma surgeons in France at that time. Broca was actually interested in language from the anthropological point of view. He was president of the Anthropological Society of Paris and he published more papers in anthropology than in aphasia. Now, Broca happened to have a patient who had a wound infection, who was also severely aphasic. People at the Salpetriere called him Tantan, because the only utterance he had was this stereotype: tantan. When he wanted to ask for a glass of water, he would say "tantantan tan tan tan", with a certain amount of gesturing and emotional prosody. When this patient died shortly after Broca examined him in detail he had the opportunity to look at the brain of this patient, the brain is still preserved in the Dupuytren museum in Paris. Interesting historical aside, that it was lost during the war because they put the museum pieces in the basement and after the war they could not find it for a long time. Eventually, an American historian uncovered the brain, but still they have not yet cut it, but they CAT-scanned it![17]. The CAT scan of Tantan's brain looked like this modern composite of persisting Broca's aphasia localization from my laboratory (Fig. 1). Patients who have a chronic persisting Broca's aphasia have, as a rule, lesions that go beyond Broca's area. Broca emphasized the frontal lesion, but when Pierre Marie drew the side view of Tantan's brain 40 years later, he said that the frontal lobe is involved, but so is the parietal lobe and he put a probe inside and found that the subcortical regions were also destroyed. In fact, Pierre Marie was right, but not when he said, "The frontal lobe has nothing to do with articulated speech". Patients who

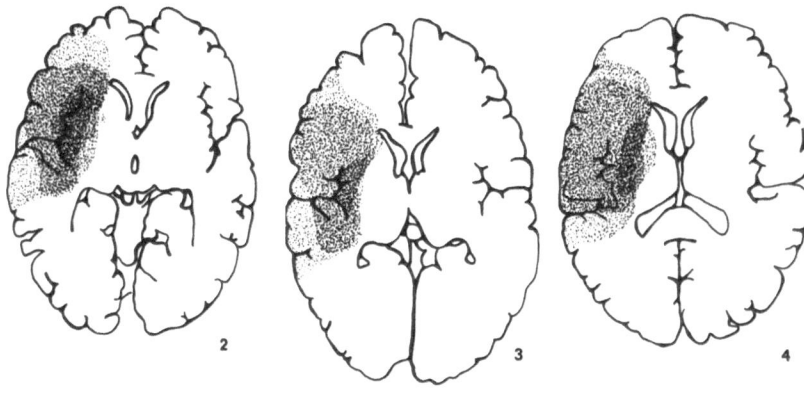

CHRONIC BROCA'S

Fig. 1. The overlap of lesions of patients who had persisting Broca's aphasia one year after the onset of stroke. (Reprinted with permission, Kertesz, Harlock and Coates, 1979). Not only Broca's area but the inferior central region and inferior parietal lobule are also involved

have only frontal lobe lesions, also have Broca's aphasia transiently. On the other hand, patients who have frontal, central and subcortical lobe lesions recover poorly. The large lesions associated with persisting Broca's aphasia often involve 3 major areas: the posterior frontal, inferior central and anterior subcortical network of articulatory mechanisms of language. In a study[9] where we collected all our chronic Broca's aphasics, we took the overlap of lesions and it corresponds to this area on the CT template, which involves not only Broca's area, but also the inferior pre- and post-central gyrus and the inferior parietal lobule (Fig. 1).

Not all Broca's aphasics have Broca's area involved. This example of a Broca's aphasia (according to the test scores on the Western Aphasia Battery [WAB]) is classified as Broca's aphasia but, Broca's area is clearly spared (Fig. 2). There is , however, a sub-cortical lesion that is striatocapsular. Ever since we have had CAT scans, we became aware of subcortical regions as, indeed, causing aphasic syndromes. Some investigators proclaim that these aphasic syndromes are atypical[14] but this is very subjective, depending on what kind of aphasia test you use and what kind of definition you have for aphasia type. The fact remains that these patients indeed, looked like a typical Broca's aphasia.

Mild motor aphasics recovering Broca's aphasics may show a particular articulatory disturbance which, in America, is often called verbal apraxia and in Europe the term "Pure Motor Aphasia" is used. These patients have a rather pure disturbance with articulatory language without any comprehension or syntactic deficit. The major problem is with initial

consonants, with consonant clusters, and it is diagnostic that the disturbance is inconsistent, meaning that sometimes they pronounce the same target, sometimes they cannot. This serves as a clear distinction from dysarthria where the slurring, omission or alteration is always the same. Verbal apraxia is frequently seen with subcortical lesions and sometimes with purely Broca's area lesions. The prognosis is good and these patients are often favored by therapists.

Several years ago, we did PET studies looking for diaschisis in recovering patients, and we found that not only the affected frontal Broca's area was hypometabolic which is what one would expect, but considerably more posterior areas remained by hypometabolic. In other words, hypometabolism persists much longer than one would expect on the basis of excellent clinical recovery. This remains controversial because some Italian and French investigations found that some of this hypometabolic region shrinks during recovery. I think this needs to be looked at very carefully. It is difficult to do repeated metabolic studies because of the expense, and the radiation involved.

A large lesion that involves both Broca's and Wernicke's areas, usually results in a devastating global aphasia. This is a similar deficit to hemispherectomies, (I do not think too many neurosurgeons do this any more, but for a while it was done for gliomas). The frontal and posterior parietal and temporal regions are damaged in the whole middle cerebral artery distribution, and areas that may compensate for language are destroyed. In adults, the right hemisphere cannot compensate, therefore, global aphasia is the consequence. However, there are exceptions, and not all large lesions will produce persisting global aphasia. We had one patient who has recovered in three months, to only a slight anomic aphasia and he was discharged from the hospital with very functional speech. The reason for this kind of expection may be found in differences in the cerebral organization of language. This patient was ambidextrous, and it is very likely that he had considerable language capacity in the right hemisphere. Another interesting case, where recovery occurred in a patient who has initially global aphasic, had central sparing. The combination of the posterior lesions and the anterior lesions can produce global aphasia, but if there is a substantial central sparing between them, it is a good prognostic sign. The central cortical tissue was able to compensate for the articulatory disturbance and for the initial comprehension disturbance. So, this particular double lesion which sometimes happens in middle cerebral embolic

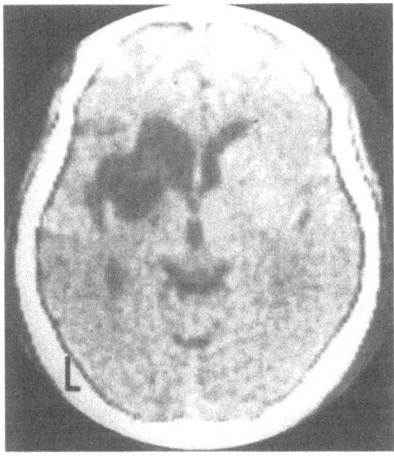

Fig. 2. Mainly subcortical lesion with Broca's aphasia. "Broca's area" is spared

strokes carries a good prognosis for recovery even though the initial deficit is severe.

The smallest lesion we found that produced a complete global aphasia, which was persisting, did not affect Broca's area, and it did not affect Wernicke's area either. A subcortical white matter infarct, undercutting these areas was found. Most of the lesion was in the periventricular white matter and the white matter around the frontal horns. The lesion produced a substantial disconnection of the speech areas. Naeser and others (1990)[15] found that most non-fluent patients had not only the periventricular white matter of the temporo-frontal radiation involved, but also the subcallosal radiation and the subcallosal fasciculus.

Another major type of aphasia is called fluent, or Wernicke's aphasia. This is indeed distinctive, and all of you who see aphasics will agree that these patients are quite different from the severe Broca's and global aphasics. This is an example of a patient's output which is very fluent but it does not make sense (Fig. 3). The sentence structure is recognizable, the words are separated and some of the words are preceded by adjectives. However, the nouns are often neologistic. Some jargon words may be considered a verb because it is preceded by an auxiliary or ends with an affix that indicates that it is a verb, except it is a neologistic jargon word. Before Wernicke, people talked about amnestic aphasia, but Wernicke pointed out that indeed there is a posterior brain region that elaborates comprehension and monitors speech output. Actually, some of Wernicke's ideas, such as the auditory feedback of motor output are very modern and stood the

test of time. Frank Benson and I collected all of the neologistic cases and we found that both the posterior superior temporal gyrus and the supramarginal gyrus have to be involved to produce jargon aphasia[8].

Our more recent studies of recovery from Wernicke's aphasia tried to determine what is really Wernicke's area? What do you really need to compensate for recovery and what lesions are seen in persisting Wernicke's aphasia? The argument of what is Wernicke's area has been a lively one and so far we have not had unequivocal data. The reasons are several; one of them is the methodology as defining what is Wernicke's aphasia is variable and the second is that the CAT scan methodology has been primitive. Our CAT methodology is based on lesion analysis by anatomical criteria by independent raters and a computer digitizing of the lesion area. In other words, we are not only looking at lesion size, but we are also looking at the extent of each anatomical structure involved. We subdivided our patient to good, moderate, and poor recovery groups. The results of the statistical analysis indicated that the most important difference between those aphasics who recover reasonably well and those who do not, is the involvement of the supramarginal and angular gyrus region. We believe that compensation in severe Wernicke's aphasia occurs in the posterior surrounding cortex. Now, this is not a cortex that is taking over function vicariously, without ever having been associated with language function. It is much more likely that these cortical structures belong to a network of language cortex that has been participating previously in the elaboration of some of language function and it has the plasticity to compensate. We found that an anterior extension in the insula and the post-central gyrus are not crucial for compensation and found that in contrast to Broca's and global aphasia where subcortical involvement is considerable, in Wernicke's aphasia it is not necessary nor is it common.

We concluded from our recovery studies that initial severity and lesion size are good predictors of recovery. Therefore, a good measure of initial severity, such as the WAB, provides a prognosis to the patients and if you have an opportunity to measure lesion size, you will increase your prognostic accuracy.

There are patients who have a disconnection between Wernicke's and Broca's area and this produces conduction aphasia. Their spontaneous speech is almost normal, apart from occasional paraphasic errors, and their comprehension is quite good. When they are asked to repeat however, they become very paraphasic.

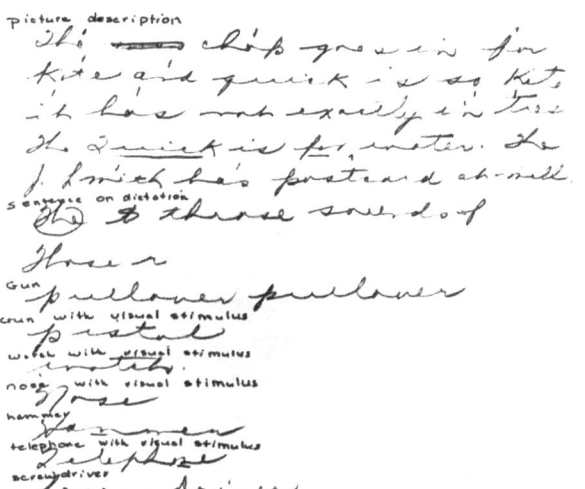

Fig. 3. Jargon agraphia from a Wernicke's aphasic

If you ask them to name, they may approximate the target words phonetically. For example, you show them a fork and then they say, "It is a bork, cork, stork, *fork*". Eventually, they may get it, or may pass the target and produce another paraphasic response. This is called the "conduit d'approche" in the French literature. These patients recover well. The majority of them will have a lesion in the posterior parietal operculum, involving the arcuate fasciculus, which conducts the input from the temporal lobe across the Sylvian fissure forward to the frontal lobe. Wernicke thought initially that much of language elaboration occurs through the insula, but Benson et al. (1983)[1] have found lesions in conduction aphasia which are entirely in the white matter. More recent MRI studies indicate that either insular, or white matter lesions are present.

The echolalic aphasic who does not understand, but has fluent speech output and repeats well is called transcortical sensory aphasia. For many years transcortical sensory aphasia was considered to be a non-localizable entity[4]. The reason for this is, that some of the patients with the transcortical sensory aphasia syndrome have Alzheimer's disease. They put out semantic jargon, they do not comprehend, but they repeat very well. These Alzheimer patients are said to be "echolalic". We discovered that, in addition, patients with posterior cerebral artery strokes also have lesions that produce transcortical sensory aphasia. Sometimes neurosurgical patients who have tentorial herniation and compress the posterior cerebral artery may end up with transcortical sensory aphasia and they may have visual agnosia as well. The lesions in our study overlapped in the watershed area between the occipital lobe and the temporal lobe (Fig. 4). Wernicke's area itself was not affected.

Transcortical motor aphasia is similar in that repetition is preserved, but the patient is nonfluent in spontaneous speech. Professor Kornyey (1975) contributed important work to show that this entity is often seen in tumors and in strokes of the supplementary motor area. It is seen frequently after anterior cerebral artery occlusion, also, especially if the occlusion involves the left mesial aspect of the frontal lobe. Bilateral involvement produces an abulic patient who not only does not talk, but does not even want to move, and a very severe variety of this is called akinetic mutism. This may be seen after anterior cerebral-anterior communicating artery aneurysm rupture. Therefore, transcortical motor aphasia is often a neurosurgical entity.

Finally, mixed transcortical patients have frontal and posterior lesions. This was also called isolation of the speech area by Goldstein and the best example with localization was described by Geschwind et al. (1968)[3]. This was a carbon monoxide victim who was considered totally aphasic, who did not speak or understand. One day, the nurses noted that this patient was singing along with the radio and they became very excited about it. When a more detailed examination was done, it was shown that this patient could repeat, but that was the only thing she could do. The patchy widespread lesions isolated the speech area, hence the term "isolation syndrome".

To end with a quote from Aristotle: "We must start by observing a set of similar individuals and consider what elements they have in common. To define and divide one need not know the whole of existence". We have looked at a representative population of 365 aphasics, and the percentages are broken down in the Table 1. These are acute stroke patients as well as neurosurgical patients. The most numerous ones are anomic, then global and Broca's aphasics and Wernicke's aphasics about equal, conduction, transcortical motor and transcortical sensory aphasics are much less frequent and the isolation syndrome is rather rare. These

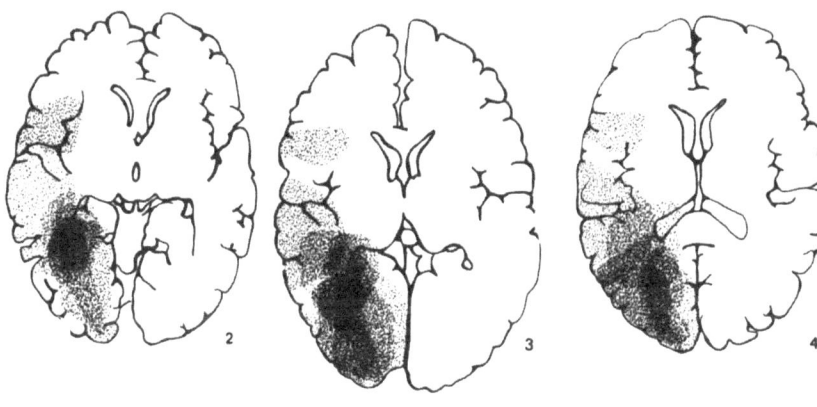

ACUTE TRANSCORTICAL
SENSORY

Fig. 4. The overlap of lesions for transcortical sensory aphasia. Reproduced with permission from Kertesz, Sheppard MacKenzie, 1982

Table 1. *Clinical Forms of Aphasia*

Global	16%
Broca's	17%
Wernicke's	15%
Anomic	29%
Conduction	9%
Transcortical motor	4%
Transcortical sensory	7%
Isolation	3%

The percentages are obtained from combining infarcts (n = 141) with a neurosurgical group (trauma and tumor, n = 74).

percentages change from the acute to the chronic syndromes and this reflects recovery patterns. This basic classification system is a useful guide for the clinician and can be a reliable tool for the researcher.

To conclude briefly a current view of localization of aphasic syndromes: for Wernicke's aphasia or fluent aphasia with comprehension deficit the superior posterior temporal lesion is obligatory, and a persisting jargon aphasia will involve the supramarginal gyrus. Broca's aphasia is, indeed, seen with posterior inferior frontal lesions, but a central and subcortical component is involved in persisting deficit, not just Broca's area. The lesions producing transcortical motor aphasia involve the supplementary speech area of Penfield and transcortical sensory aphasia have lesions that overlap the watershed area between the middle cerebral and posterior cerebral arteries. One has to keep in mind, nevertheless, the dictum of Jackson (1878)[5]: "To locate the damage which destroys speech and to localize speech are two different things".

References

1. Benson F, Sheremata WA, Bouchard R, Segara JM *et al* (1973) Conduction aphasia. Arch Neurol 28: 339–346

2. Broca P (1861) Remarques sur le siége de la faculté du language articulé, suives d'une observation d'aphemie (perte de la parole). Bull Soc Anat (Paris) 36: 330–357

3. Geschwind N, Quadfasel F, Segarra J (1968) Isolation of the speech area. Neuropsychologia 6: 327–340

4. Henschen SE (1920–1922) Klinische und anatomische Beiträge zur Pathologie des Gehirns, Vols 5–7. Stockholm, Nordiska Bokhandel

5. Jackson HJ (1878) On affections of speech from disease of the brain. Brain 1: 304–330

6. Kertesz A (1979) Aphasia and associated disorders: Taxonomy, localization and recovery. Grune & Stratton, New York

7. Kertesz A (1982) The Western Aphasia Battery. Grune & Stratton, New York

8. Kertesz A, Benson (1970) Neologistic jargon – a clinicopathological study. Cortex 6: 362–386

9. Kertesz A, Harlock W, Coates R (1979) Computer tomographic localization, lesion size and prognosis in aphasia. Brain and Lang 8: 34–50

10. Kertesz A, Sheppard A, MacKenzie R (1982) Localization in transcortical sensory aphasia. Arch Neurol 39: 475–478

11. Környey E (1975) Aphasie transcorticale et echolalie: le problème de l'initiative de la parole. Rev Neurol (Paris) 131A: 347–363

12. Marie P (1906) Revision de la question de l'aphasie: La troisième circonvolution frontale gauche ne joue aucun role special dans la fonction du language. Sem Med 21: 241–247, May 23

13. Marie P, Foix C (1917) Les aphasies de guerre. Rev Neurol (Paris) 24: 53–87

14. Naeser MA, Alexander MP, Helm-Estabrooks N, Levine HL, Laughlin SA, Geschwind N (1982) Aphasia with predominantly subcortical lesion sites. Arch Neurol 39: 2–14

15. Naeser MA, Palumbo CL, Helm-Estabrooks N, Stiassny-Eder D, Albert ML (1989) Severe non-fluency in aphasia: role of the subcallosal fasciculus and other white matter pathways in recovery or speech output. Brain 112: 1–38

16. Porch BE (1971) The Porch index of communicative ability: Administration, scoring and interpretation. Consulting Psychologists, Palo Atlo, CA

17. Signoret J-L, Castaigne P, Lhermitte F, Abelanet R, Lavoral P (1984) Rediscovery of Leborgne's brain: anatomical description with CT scan. Brain and Lang 22: 303–319

Correspondence: A. Kertesz, Department of Clinical Neurological Sciences, St. Joseph's Hospital, 268 Grosvenor St. London, Ontario, N6A 4V2, Canada.

Acta Neurochirurgica (1993) [Suppl] 56: 59–66

Aphasia in Bilinguals

B. Ramamurthi and **P. Chari**

V.H.S. Medical Centre, Madras, India

Summary

The neurophysiological and the neurolinguistic basis of multilingualism is not yet fully elucidated. A study of the occurrence of aphasia in multilingual patients and the pattern of recovery may help to clarify some unsolved problems. For e.g. is the ability to use a second language stored in a different area of the left hemisphere and what is the extent of involvement of the right hemisphere in language skills? When recovery from aphasia occurs, what factors determine the rate of recovery of different languages and the priorities of recovery?

To understand some of the problems, a study of aphasia in multilinguals was conducted in Madras, South India, where multilingualism is common. 88 patients were studied with 40 healthy controls, using standard protocols. It was found that the pattern of recovery was dispersed widely in time, rate, level, degree and between the languages known. No support was obtained for the notion that the patients' mother tongue recovers first, nor was support found for the importance of language proficiency viewed globally. Evidence was found that the languages in which routine thinking, mental calculations and praying were carried out were the ones most resistant to damage in brain insults. It is interesting that these functions are all highly overlearned, acquired early in life and used frequently over the course of many years.

Another observation made was that the incidence of crossed aphasia was fairly high, in both uni- and multi-linguals, with the latter showing a slightly higher incidence. The more than expected higher incidence of crossed aphasia in unilinguals suggests that the language capacities of the right hemisphere in unilinguals may have been underestimated in earlier literature.

There are many aspects of language function in multilingual aphasics which have to be elucidated and further extensive neurolinguistic research is necessary, before positive conclusions can be arrived at.

Keywords: Aphasia; bilinguals; multilingualism.

Introduction

A study of the occurrence of aphasia and the pattern of language recovery in bilingual aphasics is indeed intriguing and exciting, with large possibilities of contributing to our knowledge about language acquisition, comprehension, delivery and also about the role of the two hemispheres in these processes.

Since the time Broca enunciated that the faculty of language in humans was located in the left hemisphere, neurologists have been keenly interested in language function and also in the different types of dysphasia. The possible sites of localisation of different linguistic functions in different areas of the left hemisphere were worked out methodically, and naturally all these studies were in people who spoke only one language.

When a person is capable of speaking more than one language and gets afflicted with aphasia, many interesting problems arise and these had provoked keen interest even in the last half of the previous century[1,16,17]. Are both languages lost in these patients or do they lose the faculty of speech in only one of them? Is there a differential loss in the linguistic capacity? When recovery occurs, which language returns first, or do both return simultaneously? If the capacity to speak one language recovers first, which is this language? Is it the mother tongue, is it the language learned later, is it the language that has been most used by the patient, or is it the one most useful for the patient? Or do different languages return according to the need of the occasion, like emotional need, intellectual need or the need for survival?

Early Work

From a thorough study of a few bilingual patients with aphasia, Ribot in 1881 and Pitres in 1890 enunciated a few rules that appear to govern the pattern of recovery from aphasia in bilinguals. These can be summarised:

1. In multilingual aphasia, the patient does not necessarily lose the use of all languages to an equal extent.
2. When recovering, the patient first begins to understand and then to speak the language most familiar

to him. Later he recovers the use of the other languages.

3. This is possible as the language centres have only been shattered and not destroyed by the lesion.
4. The temporary inertia of the cortical language centres accounts for this sequence of phenomena and it is not necessary to assume different centres for different languages.

Since then, these rules have been quoted by many workers in the field who however noted that there were some patients who did not obey these rules[8,14]. It was obvious that there was a need to study the problem further and try to explain the different types of loss and recovery of language functions in multilinguals.

Increasing Multilingualism

In the modern world, with its easy communications and travel, learning of two or more languages has become common and the problem of multilingual aphasia was no more just esoteric but one that may affect many people in many countries. Neurolinguists, psycholinguists and neurologists have interested themselves in this study since the past three decades and a number of papers have been published about the problem of bilingualism both in healthy adults and in brain-damaged patients[24].

Degrees of Bilingualism. What is Bilingualism?

The term bilingualism itself seems to present some problems. Though bilingualism implies the ability to converse in two languages, all bilinguals are not equally proficient in both the languages. Some of them may be able to read and write both the languages, while some may be able to read and write only one of them. In some countries, it is common to find people who can converse well in two or more languages, but are unable to read or write any of them. It is apparent that there are degrees of bilingualism and when determining the rate and type of recovery from aphasia, it is necessary to have information on the degree and the type of proficiency of the patient in the languages before the brain insult.

"Co-Ordinate" and "Compound" Bilinguals

Some of the factors that determine proficiency in the *second language and* influence the rate of recovery after brain insult are the *age* at which the second

language is learnt, the *environment* in which it is learnt and the *method* by which the second language has been taught. When both the languages are learnt in early childhood by living in the environment, (compound bilingualism, Erwin and Osgood 1954) the process of language acquisition becomes much easier. In such cases the intonation and the pronunciation are as near each language as possible. When the second language is learnt later in school (coordinate bilingualism), the grammar, syntax and sentence construction etc. are much better, but the accent of the original language is likely to persist. During language recovery after brain insult, coordinate bilinguals seem to have a better chance of recovering the second language, but many other factors come into play and influence recovery.

Multifactorial

When there is a loss of language after a cerebral insult, a large number of factors come into play to determine how much language is lost and also to determine the rate and type of recovery in each language. It has been noted that even when there is equal fluency in both the languages the recovery pattern seems to be determined by many factors. One would expect that the mother tongue would be the first to recover and recover well. However our experience and experience from cases reported in the literature show that language recovery may differ in different areas of need. The usual pattern is for the recovery of language that has been most commonly used by the patient before the attack.

Background of Present Research

In Madras, South India, where this research has been conducted, the language of the people is Tamil, but most educated people use English as the language of communication. In addition to these, children and adults are exposed to the language of adjacent states namely Telugu, Kannada and Malayalam. Thus there is a fairly vast population which is multilingual. Generally this population will be able to speak, read and write the Tamil language as well as English. They may be able to speak the other languages fluently but may not be able to read and write them.

The interesting feature in the Indian context is that the educated Indian speaks the mother tongue at home for all needs and emotional purposes, using English for higher scientific thinking and official contact. Often he may use a different language (Sanskrit) for praying. It has been shown by our work that the language faculty recovers to fulfill the needs as indicated above. The pattern shows the recovery of Tamil for emotional purposes, English for intellectual purposes and the language used for praying. Hence it is obvious that apart from the length of knowledge of the language and its fluency, the need of the organism to cope with the environment often determines the pattern of recovery.

Materials and Methods

A group of 88 patients with aphasic disorders was studied using 40 healthy controls. The aphasic disorder was diagnosed on the basis of an aphasia test battery developed by Chary (1980). The aphasics ranged in age from 7 to 70 years and included 60 males and 28 females. The aetiology of the lesion was cerebrovascular in 46, head injury in 25 and space-occupying lesions in 17.

Both the controls and the aphasic subjects were classified as multilingual or unilingual. Multilinguality implied the comprehension and delivery of more than one language with near equal fluency. Literacy in the language (the ability to read or write) was not considered essential to consider a person multilingual.

Incidence of Multilingualism

Of the 88 aphasics 31 (or 35%) were multilingual (21 men and 10 women) and 57 were monolingual. Of the 40 healthy controls, 16 (40%) were multilingual and 24 (60%) were monolingual.

Table 1 shows the nature of the lesion causing the aphasia in multilinguals and monolinguals.

Table 1. *Aetiology of Lesion*

Type of injury	Multilingual aphasics (31)		Monolingual aphasics (57)	
	No.	% Total	No.	% Total
Cerebrovascular	15	48	31	54
Head injury	12	39	13	23
Tumour	4	13	13	23

Table 2 shows the age of the patients.

Table 2. *Age of Patients*

Age (years)	Multilingual aphasics (31) No.	Monolingual aphasics (57) No.
0–20	4	8
21–40	10	11
41–60	16	29
61–80	1	9

Range of Languages Known and Context of Acquisition

With the exception of one Telugu-speaking monolingual, the remaining monolinguals were all Tamil speakers. Languages known by the bilingual controls, in decreasing order, were Tamil/English, English/Tamil, and English/Telugu.

In 22 of the 31 multilingual aphasics, either all or the first two languages were acquired in a common environment (compound bilingualism). In the remaining 9 patients they were acquired under different environmental conditions (or coordinate bilingualism).

Language of the Environment

Languages used in the patient's larger environment (e.g., languages spoken by neighbours, servants, shopkeepers, etc.) are listed in Table 3, for the patients belonging to the compound bilingual subgroup.

Incidence of Literacy

Among the monolingual aphasics, 20 only of the 57 patients (35%) were literate; among the multilingual aphasics, the incidence of literacy was much higher, being 61%.

Occurrence of Language Mixing

The high incidence of code-switching and code-mixing characterising bilingual communities such as those found in India (see Sridhar 1978) makes it difficult to segregate the languages completely according to functional domain. Intrasentential language mixing is particularly prevalent among Tamil, Telugu, and English, and forms part of the day-to-day speech of this population.

Functions Served by Each Language

Language used among the multilinguals was categorized into five functional domains:

1. for daily conversation,
2. at work,
3. for routine thinking,
4. for prayer, and
5. for mental arithmetic.

Information about the multilingual patients' premorbid language use was obtained either from the patients themselves or from their relatives. Details are given in Table 4.

Table 3. *Language of Environment and Language Background*

Language background	No.	Language of environment
Tamil/English	10	Tamil/English
Telugu/English	9	Telugu/English
Tamil/Telugu	4	Tamil
Telugu/Tamil/English	4	Telugu
Tamil/English/Hindustani	1	Tamil
Kannada/English/Tamil	1	Kannada
Malayalam/Tamil/English	2	Malayalam

Table 4. *Language Used for Various Functions by the 31 Multilingual Dysphasics as Elicited from the Patients, Their Relatives and on Recovery from Dysphasia*

Nature of language acquisition and languages known	No. of patients	Mother tongue	Languages used				
			Daily conversation	At work	To think	To pray	To calculate
Compound language group (22)							
Tamil/English, English/Tamil and Telugu/English	10	Tamil or Telugu	Tamil or Telugu and English	English and Tamil	Tamil-6 English-4	Tamil-8 English-2	Tamil-9 English-1
Tamil/Telugu	4	Tamil	Tamil	English and Tamil	Tamil	Tamil	Tamil
Telugu/Tamil/ English	4	Telugu	Telugu	English Tamil and Telugu	Telugu-3 Telugu and English-1	Telugu	Telugu
Tamil/English/ Hindustani	1	Tamil	Tamil	English and Tamil	Tamil and English	Tamil	Tamil
Kannada/English/ Tamil	1	Kannada	Kannada	English and Tamil	Kannada	Kannada	Kannada
Malayalam/Tamil/ English	2	Malayalam	Malayalam	English and Tamil	Malayalam and English	Malayalam	Malayalam
Coordinate language group (9)							
Tamil/English and English/Tamil	5	Tamil	Tamil	English and Tamil	Tamil	Tamil	Tamil
Tamil/Telugu	2	Tamil	Tamil	English and Tamil	Tamil	Tamil	Tamil
Telugu/English	1	Telugu	Telugu	English	Telugu	Telugu	Telugu
Hindustani/Tamil/ English	1	Tamil	Hindustani	English and Tamil	Hindustani	Hindustani	Hindustani

Neuropsychological Assessment

All subjects were administered a core aphasia test battery (Chary 1980), with some additional tests devised to accommodate the particular characteristics (e.g. illiteracy, multi- or bilingualism) etc. of the population under study. After a complete neurological examination and assessment of cortical functions, the handedness was determined and language and cognitive functions evaluated. Information was gathered about free conversation, contextual conversation, auditory perception, visual comprehension and perception, somatic and spatial orientation, speech formulation, drawing and copying and reading and writing. Tests were also incorporated to detect apraxia, agnosia and their influence on speech disorder (Tables 5 and 6).

Table 5. *Evaluation of Language and Other Cognitive Functions*

1. Free conversation.	9. Serial and sequential integration
2. Contextual conversation	10. Somatic orientation
3. Auditory perception	11. Spatial orientation and integration
4. Repetition	
5. Series recitation	12. Numerical and topographical relationships
6. Simple speech formulation	
7. Complex speech formulation	13. Drawing and copying
8. Visual comprehension and perception	14. Reading and writing

Table 6. *Linguistic Analysis to Detect Errors in Speech*

a) Phonological level
   i. articulator errors
   ii. phonemic errors
b) Syntactic
   i. errors of omission
   ii. paragrammatic errors
c) Semantic context
   i. conceptual (denotative meaning)
   ii. perceptual (connotative meaning)

Overall
i. defect in comprehension
ii. defect in production

From all the above observations, a clinical localisation was arrived at and then validated by other measures like angiogram, C.T., and operation when indicated.

Results

It may be noted that all the three coordinate bilinguals improved, whereas only 10 out of 17 compound multilinguals showed improvement.

Table 7. *Follow-up in Multilingual Dysphasics*

Multilingual patients	31
two died	nine drop outs
Followed-up	20 patients

Table 8. *Follow-up in Multilingual Dysphasics*

	20	
	followed-up	
co-ordinate (3)		compound (17)
all improved		
improved	stationary	deteriorated
10	6	1

Table 9. *Incidence of Crossed Aphasia*

Number of patients	Handedness	Side of lesion		
		Left	Right	Diffuse/ bilateral
57 Monolinguals	right (52)	34	5	13
	left (5)	2	1	2
31 Multilinguals	right (27)	19	3	5
	left (4)	2	2	0

A detailed analysis of the improvement pattern supported the following observations. When considering the overall performance of the multilingual aphasics who were followed up, the following generalisations were supported.

1. The pattern of language recovery was dispersed widely in time, rate, level, degree and between languages known.
2. When task-oriented languages were considered, the following consistent patterns were noted.
   (a) In the patients who improved, the language which recovered first and/or best was that used for routine thinking and calculations. This language was not necessarily the patient's mother tongue.
   (b) Among patients who reported thinking mainly in one language (e.g., English) but who performed mental arithmetic in another language (e.g., Tamil) the language used for mental calculations was the one that recovered first.
   (c) Among patients whose languages deteriorated over time, the language used for praying was retained the longest.

The incidence of crossed aphasia was fairly high, in both unilinguals and multilinguals with multilinguals showing a slightly higher incidence.

There are two noteworthy findings from the present study. The first concerns patterns of language impairment and/or recovery in polygot aphasia. The second concerns the role of the right hemisphere in normal language processing.

No support was obtained for the notion that the patient's mother tongue recovers first nor was support found for the importance of language proficiency viewed globally. Specifically, evidence was found that the languages in which routine thinking, mental calculations, and praying occur were the ones that were more resistant to the debilitating effects of brain injury. It is interesting that these functions are all highly over-learned, acquired fairly early in life, and used frequently over the course of many years.

The other interesting finding of the present study revolves around the incidence of aphasia produced by damage to the right hemisphere. Crossed aphasia was found among a sizable percentage of the aphasics, both in unilinguals and multilinguals.

Greater right hemisphere involvement in (premorbid) language functioning in polygots than in monolinguals has previously been claimed (see Galloway 1981)[7] on the basis of predominantly single case reports gleaned from the published literature.

The present study found a remarkably high percentage of crossed aphasia among unilinguals (see Table 9). This finding suggests that the language capacities of the right hemisphere in unilinguals may have been underestimated in the literature at large.

Discussion

Observations have shown that in multilingual aphasia, recovery of the language may vary. Generally six different patterns, have been noticed: (Lecours *et al.* 1983)[12] *parallel* recovery when all the languages are restored at the same rate. This is the common type of recovery. *Differential* recovery occurs when one or more languages are recovered more slowly than others. *Successive* implies that recovery of the second language takes place only after the first language has been recovered.

In *selective* recovery one or two languages which the patient has learnt do not get restored. There may be loss of comprehension or expression in the languages.

In *antagonistic* recovery, as one language is recovering the other language regresses. In *mixed* recovery the bilinguals mix their two languages. It should be noted that mixed recovery is common among people who resort to intrasentential switching in daily language, as is most commonly obtained in the Indian population.

Many theories have been put forward to explain the differential recovery of languages. According to Ribot (1981) languages acquired in childhood are most resistant to aphasia; consequently the mother tongue will be least impaired and will be the first to recover. According to Pitres the determining factor of recovery is the degree of practice in the particular language. Thus the most commonly used language recovers first.

Minkowski (1928) proposed that psychological and emotional components determine the language that recovers. Other factors that may influence recovery, are reading and writing proficiency in the language. The other possibility is that the language which has preferentially recovered is the one which is most useful to the patient for his day-to-day needs. This is what our work has confirmed.

In any particular instance all the above factors and also the severity of the brain damage determine the ultimate recovery.

It is obvious that the factors that influence recovery are multiple and include the order in which the languages were learnt, the degree of proficiency, emotional attachment to the language, the age of the patient, his intellectual level and the degree of brain damage.

In the present work, the language used for routine thinking and calculation was found to recover first, not necessarily the mother tongue.

Different Circuits for Different Languages

Differential recovery of languages in multilingual aphasics may also suggest that the neurological centres and tracts responsible for each language may be different and the degree of involvement of each of these circuits during brain damage and their differential recovery may determine which language recovers first. This may sound simple and may explain all the different features that we see in language recovery in multilinguals. The brain with its enormous potential and reserves both in energy and in tissue may choose to enter each language in a different circuit, as it is being learnt. However positive proof for such a theory is not *yet available.* Hummel (1986) studying memory for information encoded and transmitted in two linguisti-

cally distinct channels concluded: "The present findings support a separate systems or independence view of bilingual organisation. If the underlying representations of the two languages were not to some extent separate, one would not have obtained a significant difference in performance as a function of whether information was conveyed via one language or two". On the contrary, Wulfeck *et al.* (1986) conclude "Our data indicate that bilinguals do not engage in separate modes of processing in their two languages. On the contrary, they appear to possess a unitary system which operates in the same fashion for both the languages. Further intensive work is clearly needed".

Language and the Right Hemisphere

The general understanding for many decades has been that the left hemisphere is the "dominant" one and the function of language is its responsibility. This is reinforced by the fact that right-handed people with left hemisphere lesions develop difficulty in language understanding and expression. It was also understood that in pure left-handers, the right brain took over this "dominant" role and housed the language faculties. However, there were cases in whom though it was the right brain that was involved in the insult, the language faculty was impaired (the syndrome of "crossed aphasia"), thus evoking interest in the role of the right brain in language faculties. Evidence has accumulated that the right brain plays a more important role in language learning and expression than has been suspected.

Analysis of the two hemisphere functions has shown that the mode of functioning of the left hemisphere is "analytic sequential" and of the right brain is "holistic-parallel".

The important part that the right brain plays in many essential functions of the brain is well known now and it is clear that the language faculty with all its connotations of cognition, emotion, recognition, recall and expression cannot be the preserve of the left hemisphere alone. The right brain has to get involved from infancy during the learning process and enough evidence is available now to confirm the important role played by the right hemisphere in the acquisition of the first language (Segalowitz 1979, 1983)[20,21].

Does the right hemisphere play a greater role in the acquisition of a second language by an older child or an adult? Such a greater right hemisphere involvement in the acquisition of second language by right-handed individuals has both experimental and clinical proof.

Critchley (1962) reported that individuals with right

hemisphere damage had difficulty in learning new languages. Tachistoscopic and dichotic listening studies have shown that the first language is more left lateralised in bilinguals (Gazier et al. 1977, Obler et al. 1975). This view is contradicted by other studies. These differences are probably due to the age and the circumstances under which the second language was acquired.

The various possibilities suggested about the role of the two hemispheres in bilinguals can be summed up as follows (Lecours, et al. 1983)[12]: 1) Both languages in one hemisphere (usually the left). 2) One language in the left and the other in the right. 3) One language in the left and the other in both hemispheres. 4) Both languages in both the hemispheres. Such apparently contradictory views have been proposed by various workers based on the study of particular cases. Different modes of organisation of languages may be possible in different people by the way they learn the languages, the strategies that they use (gestaltic or analytical strategies), the age of language acquisition, the circumstance of acquisition, sex, the degree of handedness, the emotional component involved etc.

Intrasentential Code-Switching

A difficult aspect of this study is the prevalence of the habit of using different languages within one sentence, "intrasentential code-switching" and to ascertain how much this influences differential language recovery in aphasics. Generally one would expect that a bilingual would use a different language depending on the person with whom he is carrying on the conversation. However in communities where two or more languages coexist, alternate use of the languages in a single situation often occurs. In fact such language switching within sentences has to be accepted as a normal practice in the community. Gumperz (1976) referred to this as conversational code-switching as opposed to situational code-switching. Such language switching in a single situation may have a deeper significance. Gal (1978) reported that in a Hungarian-German bilingual community in Austria, switching to German occurs "to strengthen, command and to assert expertise and authoritativeness on an issue or about a technical speciality". Such a situation is common in bilinguals in India, where switches to English occur for precisely the above reasons.

Sridhar and Sridhar (1980) have proposed that in intrasentential language switching there is a guest and host language, where guest elements are used in the host language, obeying the placement rules of the host language. The similarity in the rules of grammar in the Indoeuropean languages make this switching relatively easy. However this makes a study of recovery of languages in bilingual aphasics a difficult task.

Conclusion

Studying recovery of language function in multilingual aphasics is a difficult and painstaking process as many factors are involved in the recovery of the learnt languages. There is a need for standardisation of approach so that results could be compared. Further extensive neurolinguistic research is necessary using all the available modern investigative techniques of brain function, before any positive conclusions can be reached on how the brain processes various languages that are learnt and how they are affected in disease.

Acknowledgement

The authors thank Messrs, L.E.A., London and Baillière Tindal, London, for their permission to include material from the books, "Language Processing in Bilinguals" and "Aphasiology", respectively.

References

1. Albert M, Obler L (1978) The bilingual brain. Academic Press, New York
2. Chary P (1980) Speech disorders in South Indians. Doctoral dissertation, University of Madras
3. Chary P (1986) Aphasia in a multilingual society. In: Vaid J (ed) Language processing in bilinguals; psycholinguistic and neuropsychological perspectives. Lawrence Erlbaum Ass., London, pp 183–197
4. Critchley M (1962) Speech and speech loss in relation to the duality of the brain. In: Mount Castle UB (ed) Interhemispheric relations and cerebral dominance. Johns Hopkins Univ Press, Baltimore
5. Ervin S, Osgood C (1954) Second language learning and bilingualism. J Abnorm Soc Psychol 49: 139–146
6. Gal S (1978) Variation and change in patterns of speaking: Language shifts in Austria. In: Sankoff D (ed) Linguistic variation. Academic Press, New York
7. Galloway L (1981) Contribution of the right cerebral hemisphere to language and communication. Unpublished doctoral dissertation, University of California, Los Angeles
8. Gloning I, Gloning K (1965) Aphasien bei Polyglotten. Beitrag zur Dynamik des Sprachabbaus sowie zur Lokalisationsfrage dieser Störungen. Wien Z. Nervenheilk 22: 362–397
9. Graziel T, Obler L, Bentin S, Albert M (1977) The dynamics of lateralization in second language learning: Sex and proficiency effects. Paper read at Boston University Conference on Language Development, Boston, Mass
10. Gumperz J (1976) The sociolinguistic significance of conversational code-switching. Working papers of the Language Behavior Research Laboratory, #46. University of California, Berkeley
11. Hummel KM (1986) Memory for bilingual prose. In: Vaid J (ed) Language processing in bilinguals. Psycholinguistic and neuropsychological perspectives. L.E.A. Publishers, London

12. Lecours AR, Lhermittef, Bryans (1983) Aphasia in bilinguals and polyglots. In: Lecours AR, Lhermitte F, Bryans B (eds) Aphasiology. Baillere Tindall, London, pp 455–464

13. Minkowski M (1928) Sur un cas d'aphasie chez un polyglotte. Rev Neurol (Paris) 1: 36

14. Nair K, Virmani V (1973) Speech and language disturbances in hemiplegics. Indian J Med Res 61: 1395–1403

15. Obler LK, Albert M, Gordon H (1975) Asymmetry of cerebral dominance in Hebrew-English bilinguals. Paper read at Thirteenth Annual Meeting of the Academy of Aphasia, Victoria, Canada

16. Paradis M (1977) Bilingualism and aphasia. In: Whitaker H, Whitaker HA (eds) Studies in neurolinguistics, Vol 3. Academic Press, New York, pp 65

17. Paradis M (1983) Readings on aphasia in bilinguals and polyglots. Didier, Montreal

18. Pitres A (1895) Étude sur l'aphasie chez les polyglottes. Rev Med 15: 873–899

19. Ribot T (1881) Diseases of memory: An essay in the positive psychology. Paul, London

20. Segalowitz SJ (1979) Infant cerebral asymmetries and developmental models of brain lateralization. Paper read at the 40th Annual Meeting of the Canadian Psychological Association, Quebec, Canada

21. Segalowitz SJ (1983) Cerebral asymmetries for speech in infancy. In: Segalowitz SJ (ed) Language functions and brain organization Academic Press, New York, pp 221–229

22. Sridhar SN (1978) On the functions of code-mixing in Canada. Int J Soc Lang 16: 109–118

23. Sridhar S, Sridhar K (1980) The syntax and psycholinguistics of bilingual code-mixing. Can J Psychol 34: 407–416

24. Vaid J (1986) Language processing in bilinguals. Psycholinguistic and neuropsychological perspectives. L.E.A. Publishers, London

25. Wulfeck BB et al. (1986) Sentence interpretation strategies in health and aphasic bilingual adults. In: Vaid J (ed) Language processing in bilinguals. Psycholinguistic and neuropsychological perspectives. L.E.A. Publishers, London, pp 199–219

Correspondence: B. Ramamurthi, Neurosurgeon, V.H.S. Medical Centre, Madras-600113, India.

Acta Neurochirurgica (1993) [Suppl] 56: 67–71

Operations on Gliomas Involving Speech Centres

P. Tandon and **A.K. Mahapatra** in collaboration with **Anil Khosla**

Department of Neurosurgery, All India Institute of Medical Sciences, New Delhi, India

Summary

One hundred patients with gliomas of the dominant hemisphere, who survived for more than one year after operation, have been analysed. In all of them radical tumour removal had been attempted. Already preoperatively 58 of them had signs of speech deficit. Postoperatively 65% improved and only 15% deteriorated with regard to their speech function.

Therefore it seems not to be justified to deny operative tumour removal to patients with gliomas located within or near the speech areas.

Keywords: Glioma surgery; eloquent area; speech area; results.

Introduction

With all its limitations, "radical" surgical removal of supratentorial hemisphere gliomas is now generally recognised as a desirable approach for their management. However, even amongst those who advocate surgical extirpation of such tumours, serious reservations are expressed regarding tumours involving the speech areas, for fear of producing or exacerbating an existing speech defect. Thus Pasztor (1980)[5], while advocating surgery for these tumours stated, "we do not operate when the central region, *the area of Broca and Wernicke Centre,* or when the deep midline structures are infiltrated". Garfield (1986)[2] commented that "traditionally, severe and distressing focal deficit, such as aphasia has been regarded as a contraindication to attempts at tumour removal". Such opinions persist in spite of the fact that as early as 1935, Zollinger noted that even hemispherectomy of the dominant hemisphere for gliomas did not abolish, but severely restricted speech. This was later confirmed by Basser (1962) and Smith and Burklund (1966)[8] and Burklund and Smith (1977)[1].

In 1984 at the International Symposium on Biology of Brain Tumours, we presented our experience with a large series of supratentorial gliomas, highlighting the usefulness of radical surgical removal even for tumours of the dominant hemisphere[9]. A "Medlar" search for publications on this subject during the last 6 years failed to reveal any sizeable series. The present report is an extension of our earlier study, which reconfirms the validity of our earlier approach.

Material and Methods

In our Clinic, we have, as a result of a conscious decision, operated upon all patients with supratentorial hemisphere gliomas irrespective of their location and the clinical status. The present series is derived from a cohort of such patients who have been followed postoperatively for the quality and duration of survival. One hundred patients with gliomas of the dominant hemisphere who have survived for more than one year after operation, have been analysed for the purpose of this presentation.

The surgical approach was aimed at "radical" tumour removal as described by us earlier[9]. Basically it consisted of a frontal or temporal lobectomy in cases of tumours in the anterior or middle frontal, temporal lobe. Additional intratumoural decompression was done if the tumour extended posterior to the line of section. Parietal lobe tumours were approached through the superior parietal lobule. In cases where the tumour presented on the surface, intratumoural decompression, with or without additional removal of surrounding brain from non-eloquent areas, was carried out. No external decompression was ever used. In recent years CUSA, Laser and the operating microscope have been used in selected cases.

The location of these tumours as evaluated by CT scans is summarised in Table 1. Fifty-eight of them had definite evidence of involvement of speech before the operation. It was the presenting symptom in 11 cases, it developed during mid-course in 25 and late in the evolution of symptoms in 7. Fifteen patients could not provide information about this. The pre-operative and postoperative status of speech in the series as a whole is summarized in Table 2. Amongst those whose speech was normal preoperatively (36 patients) only 4 developed postoperatively some degree of dysphasia; none became aphasic. Of 54 patients who were dysphasic before operation 35 showed significant improvement in their speech one year or more after the operation. Speech deteriorated to varying extent in 11 cases and 2 became aphasic. Three out of 4 patients who were aphasic pre-operatively regained speech postoperatively, though none of them recovered normal speech. In 6 patients speech could not be

Table 1. *Speech in Left Hemispheric Glioma (Surviving More than 1 Year Postoperative)* An analysis of 100 patients

Location of glioma	No.
Frontal	37
Temporal	26
Parietal	15
Fronto-parietal	12
Fronto-temporal	5
Temporo-parietal	4
Parieto-occipital	1
	100

Table 2. *Speech Status: Pre-operative and Postoperative*

Preoperative		Postoperative		
		Same	Better	Worse
Normal	36	32	–	4
Dysphasic	54	8	35	11
Aphasic	4	1	3	–
Could not be assessed	6			
Normal	2			
Dysphasic	4*			

* Owing to difficulty in pre-operative assessment, it is not possible to state if the speech of these patients improved or remained unchanged.

evaluated pre-operatively owing to sensorial disturbances. Amongst them speech was normal in 2, while 4 had varying degrees of dysphasia postoperatively. Thus, amongst these 100 patients operated upon for supratentorial gliomas the speech remained the same as preoperatively in 41, improved in 38 and deteriorated in 15.

Illustrative Cases

Case 1

G.S. a 60-year-old man was admitted to our Unit on 10.12.1986 with one and a half months history of progressive weakness of right side of the body and difficulty in expression. On examination he was found to have expressive dysphasia and right hemiparesis. A CT scan (Fig. 1a) showed a large mixed attenuating lesion in the posterior frontal region with gross shift of the midline. A left frontal lobectomy with intratumoral decompression was carried out. Biopsy confirmed it to be a glioblastoma. During the next three weeks, the patient showed progressive recovery of his hemiparesis and dysphasia. A repeat CT scan done in November 1988 (Fig. 1b) did not show any evidence of recurrence but only changes secondary to left frontal lobectomy. However, in January 1989, the patient developed progressive right hemiparesis and expressive dyphasia. He deteriorated over the next couple of months and died two and a half years after operation.

Case 2

S.D. a 60-year-old female was admitted to our Unit with a history of generalized headache for two and a half months, progressive right

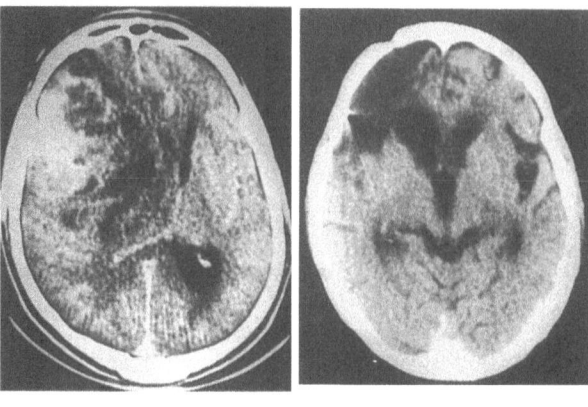

a   b

Fig. 1a, b. (a) Contrast-enhanced CT scan shows a mixed attenuating lesion in the left posterior frontal region with gross shift of the midline structures. (b) Follow up CT scan approximately two years later – no residual tumour is seen. Evidence of old frontal lobectomy is seen

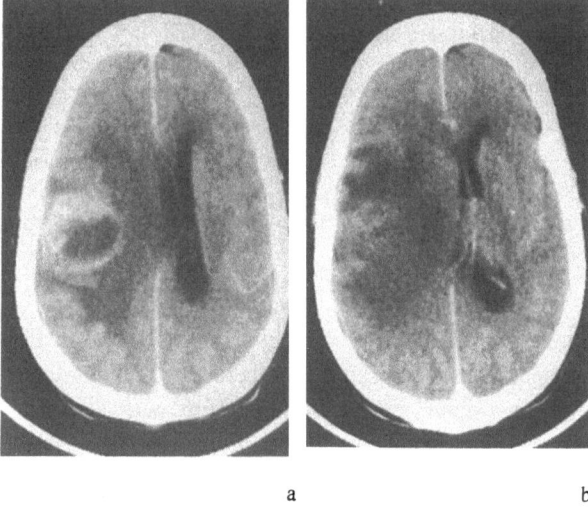

a   b

Fig. 2. Contrast-enhanced CT showing a posterior frontal-parietal tumour

hemiparesis and difficulty in speaking for two months. On examination she was found to have expressive dysphasia, with near normal comprehension. She could barely tell her name. Power in the right upper limb was 1–2/5 and lower limb 3/5. A contrast-enhanced CT scan (Fig. 2) revealed multiple irregular ring lesions in the left posterior frontal parietal area with peritumoral oedema. She was operated upon through a left posterior fronto-parietal craniotomy 4 cm away from the midline. On opening the dura the tumour was seen on the surface over a 3 cms area. The tumour was moderately vascular, solid with a small area of cystic degeneration. Microsurgical intratumoral radical decompression was performed. Postoperatively within 24 hours her speech started to show improvement. At the time of discharge from hospital on the eighth postoperative day her speech was practically normal and right-sided hemiparesis had improved (power 4–4 + /5). Histopathology confirmed that the tumour was a malignant astrocytoma.

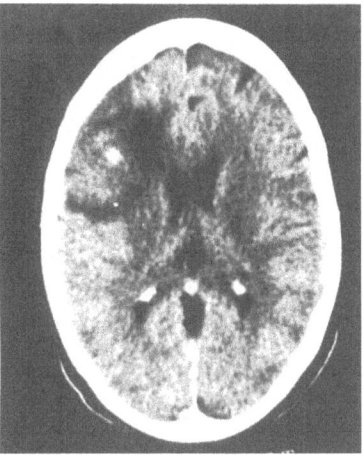

Fig. 3. Contrast-enhanced CT scan showing an isodense lesion with a small area of calcification and surrounding low attenuation in the left midfrontal region

Case 3

P.W. a 65-year-old female was admitted in October 1988, with 15 days history of progressive hemiparesis and difficulty in speaking. Three days prior to admission she developed incontinence of urine. On examination she was drowsy, had gross expressive dysphasia and she only spoke a few words. Motor power on the right side was 3/5. A contrast enhanced CT scan (Fig. 3) revealed a mixed attenuating mass with a small calcified area in the left midfrontal region. There was no significant midline shift. She was operated upon through a left frontal craniotomy and a moderately vascular tumour was radically excised. At the time of discharge from the hospital, she was still dysphasic, although her speech had improved. She was able to communicate with some difficulty. Her right hemiparesis had improved to 4–4 + /5. Histopathological examination revealed a mixed glioma. She received a full dose of radiation. A repeat CT scan in February 1989, did not show any tumour, only some postoperative

changes. At the time of her last follow-up one and a half years later she was doing well. Motor power on the right side was normal. She also had occasional difficulty in naming objects but was able to communicate reasonably well and do her day-to-day household work.

Case 4

S.M. a 45-year-old male was admitted with complaints of increasing headache for three months and altered sensorium for 15 days. On examination he was found to be grossly disoriented and had a right hemiparesis (power 4/5). Speech could not be properly evaluated. A CT scan (Fig. 4a) showed a large "cystic" tumour in the region of the trigone on the left side which displaced the choroid plexus anteriorly. A radical tumour removal was done through a parieto-temporal craniotomy. Ten days postoperatively a CT scan (Fig. 4b) showed marked reduction in the tumour bulk, reformation of the trigone and patches of blood in the tumour removal cavity. He improved progressively over next three months at which time he had only a minimal dysphasia.

Case 5

JPS. a 36-year-old male was admitted to our service in 1987 with complaints of partial complex seizures for seven months. On examination no neurological deficit was detected. A CT scan (Fig. 5a) showed a large low attenuating lesion in the left frontal opercular

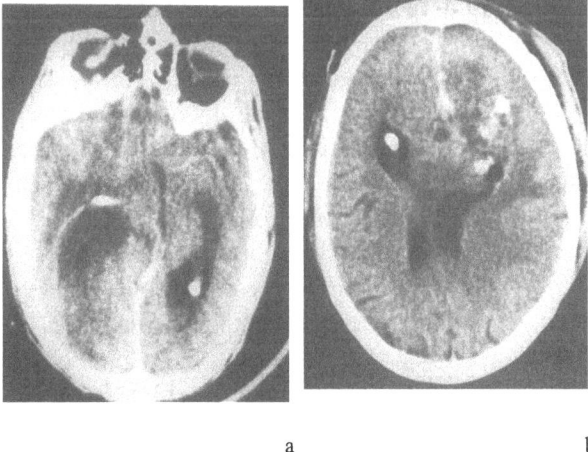

a   b

Fig. 4a, b. (a) Contrast-enhanced CT scan shows a low attenuating lesion with some enhancement at the periphery medially, in the region of the left trigone, displaying the choroid plexus anteriorly. (b) CT scan ten days after operation shows reduction of the tumour bulk

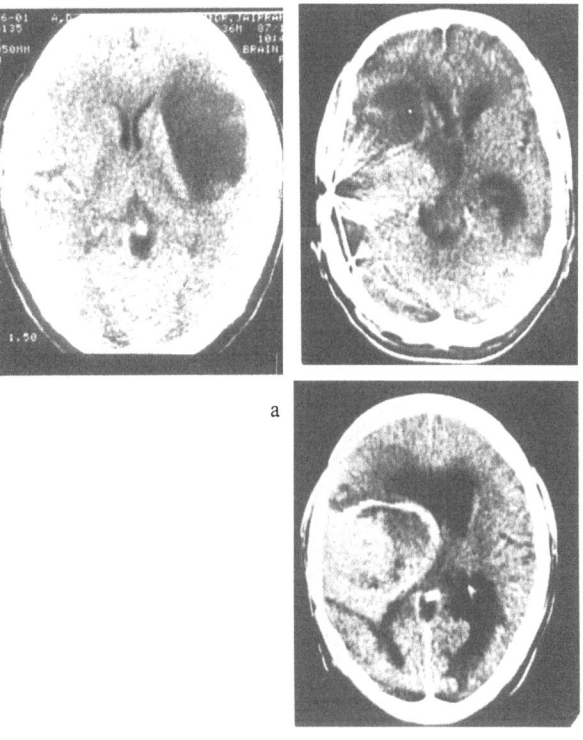

a

b

Fig. 5a, b. (a) CT scan showing a large low attenuating lesion in left opercular area. (b) CT scan two years postoperatively shows recurrence of tumour posterior to the original site of operation

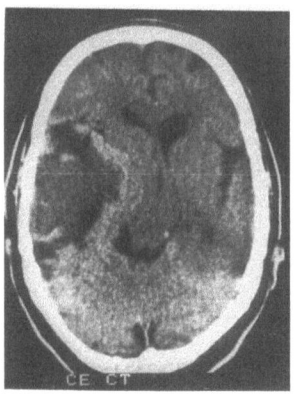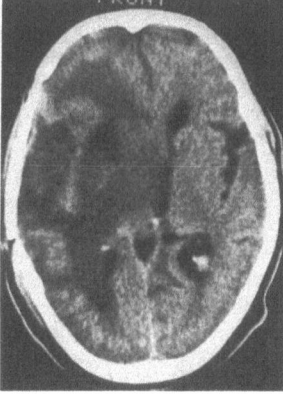

a   b

Fig. 6a, b. (a) CT scan shows a large low attenuating left fronto-temporal tumour. (b) CT scan six months postoperative

region. Surgical removal of a relatively low grade astrocytoma was performed. Immediately postoperatively he was found to be hemiplegic and aphasic. Over the next six months there was progressive improvement both in power and speech. Two years after operation the tumour recurred posterior to the original site. (Fig. 5b).

Comments: The hemiplegia and aphasia immediately after operation was very likely due to either straying outside the limits of the ill-defined tumour or undue manipulation of branches of the middle cerebral arteries in the insula which were enmeshed in the tumour. Use of the operating microscope and laser could have prevented this mishap. Nevertheless one could argue that the operation was ill-advised. It may, however, be pointed out that in spite of complete expressive dysphasia after operation, there was a significant and useful recovery of speech within six months.

Case 6

K.L. a 50-year-old male was admitted with a history of increasing headache, progressive right hemiparesis and speech difficulty for three months. Physical examination confirmed the hemiparesis (power 4/5) and a predominantly expressive dysphasia. A contrast enhanced CT scan (Fig. 6a) showed a large left frontotemporal ill-defined low-attenuating tumour with irregular peripheral enhancement. A radical surgical removal of the tumour was performed. Immediately postoperatively the hemiparesis improved but the dysphasia remained unchanged. There was a distinct improvement in the speech defect three months later. In spite of a very bizarre CT appearance (Fig. 6b), six months later, the patient had maintained good progress.

Discussion

Surgical treatment of supratentorial gliomas remains a dismal chapter in neurosurgery. It is undeniable that all modes of current therapy fail in the majority of cases to provide a cure. The aim of treatment therefore remains to prolong useful life. In spite of all advances in chemotherapy, immunotherapy, improvements in surgical techniques and radiotherapy, there is no break-*through in sight. So for the present it is generally agreed* that maximal surgical reduction in the tumour mass

followed by radiotherapy provides the best results. While this is so for tumours in the so-called non-eloquent areas of the brain, there continues to be some reservation when the tumour is in or near a vital area, for example the speech area.

In our department at the All India Institute of Medical Sciences, New Delhi, we have over the years, followed a consistent policy of surgically attacking all patients with supratentorial gliomas irrespective of the extent of pre-operative neurological deficit or the location of the tumour in the hemisphere. This procedure was adopted with the aim of establishing a histological diagnosis and reducing the tumour mass for relief of pressure symptoms. It was soon realized that the neurological deficit is often due to displacement rather than actual infiltration of the eloquent area. Furthermore, if the tumour had infiltrated vital areas and rendered them non-functional, then surgical removal, if one stays within the limit of grossly evident tumour, does not increase the neurological deficit. This attitude was obviously influenced by the senior author's training with Dr. Arthur Elvidge, who often stated, "if a tumour can go there, my finger can go there also" (implying that it would do so without adding to the damage).

The findings in the current series reiterate our earlier observations[9]. Firstly the immediate postoperative mortality and long-term survival was the same for tumours in either hemisphere. This would seem to indicate that we were able to achieve satisfactory decompression. This was further confirmed by post-operative CT scans in most of these patients. It has been observed that even when the patients had definite evidence of a speech defect pre-operatively, radical surgical removal of the tumour resulted in improvement in 38 out of 58 patients (66%), it remained the same in 9 and deteriorated in 11. Even amongst those with deterioration, there was none who developed complete aphasia. Most of them had reasonable degree of comprehension and expression to be able to carry on with at least the activities of daily living.

Most of these patients were harbouring large tumours as can be seen from the illustrative cases included here. Their CT scans revealed the tumours to be in close proximity to or actually involving either the anterior (Broca's) or the posterior (Wernicke's) speech areas. Most of the tumours, of course, extended well beyond these areas.

While attempts have been made to define the landmarks of the speech areas on a CT scan[3], it may be mentioned that in the presence of large tumours the conventional two dimension pictures fail to indicate clearly if the tumour is displacing or actually infiltrating the speech areas. A recent report by Hu *et al.* (1990) describes a method of using MR data to create three dimensional views of the brain, which make it possible to assess the spatial relationship of a lesion to the motor, sensory or speech areas. With the aid of this technique, the surgeon might be able to anticipate the difficulty in removing the lesion without sacrificing the movement, sensation, hearing and speech functions.

The present series demonstrates the feasibility of achieving major decompression using only the conventional methods of diagnosis and operation. No doubt this resulted in improvement or status quo in the majority of cases, however the ultimate aim should be either to achieve improvement in all or to be able to determine pre-operatively those who would not improve and even more so who are likely to deteriorate. Our recent experience with the use of the operating microscope, CUSA and Laser suggests that these adjuncts to surgery help to reduce the number of those who suffer deterioration. Shapiro (1982)[7] observed that the "resection of neuroectodermal tumours is more likely to alleviate existing symptoms than to produce additional ones". Salcman (1985)[6] supported this observation stating "It is now possible to safely remove large glial tumours from virtually any hemispheric-location without significant impairment of the patient". Undoubtedly if the tumour has infiltrated and irrevocably destroyed a large part of the speech area surgical decompression cannot be expected to result in improvement. The experience of Burklund and Smith (1977)[1] whose patients improved in spite of a complete hemispherectomy, raises hopes even for such patients.

Conclusions

Even with the availability of CT scans it is not possible to determine pre-operatively if a tumour in the region of the speech area is producing speech defect by compression, displacement or actual infiltration. The results of the present series demonstrate that 65 per cent of patients with clinical evidence of speech impairment pre-operatively showed unequivocal evidence of improvement after radical surgical decompression of gliomas situated in and around the speech area. These results are likely to improve with routine use of laser and CUSA.

As long as surgical reduction of the tumour mass remains a desirable goal of management of gliomas, the authors do not find any justification for denying it to those with lesions producing a speech defect.

References

1. Burklund CW, Smith A (1977) Language and cerebral hemispheres. Neurology 27: 627–633
2. Garfield JS (1987) Malignant intracranial tumours. In: Miller JD (ed) Northfield's surgery of the central nervous system, 2nd Ed. Blackwell, Oxford, pp 178–227
3. Hayward RW, Naeser MA, Zatz LM (1977) Cranial computed tomography in aphasia. Radiology 123: 653–660
4. Hu X, Tan KK, Levin DN, Galhotra S, Mullan JF, Hekmatpanah J, Spire JP (1990) Three-dimensional magnetic resonance images of the brain: Application to neurosurgical planning. J Neurosurg 72: 433–440
5. Pasztor E (1980) Hemispheric intracerebral tumours. In: Concise neurosurgery for general practitioners and students. Akade'miai Kiado', Budapest, pp 62
6. Salcman M (1985) Supratentorial gliomas: Clinical features and surgical therapy. In: Wilkin RH, Rengachery SS (eds) Neurosurgery, Vol 1. McGraw Hill, New York, pp 579
7. Shapiro WR (1982) Treatment of neuroectodermal brain tumours. Ann Neurol 12: 231–237
8. Smith A, Burklund CW (1966) Dominant hemispherectomy, preliminary report on neuropsychological sequelae. Science 153: 1280–1282
9. Tandon PN, Agarwal SP, Mahapatra AK, Roy S (1986) "Radical" surgical decompression of supratentorial gliomas. Do the results justify operation? In: Walker MD, Thomas DGT (eds) Biology of brain tumours. Martinus Nijhoff, Boston, pp 277

Correspondence: P. Tandon, Department of Neurosurgery, All India Institute of Medical Sciences, Ansari Nagar, New Delhi 110029, India.

Acta Neurochirurgica (1993) [Suppl] 56: 72–82

The Surgery for Epilepsy with Speech Arrest

C.B.T. Adams

Department of Neurosurgery, Radcliffe Infirmary, Oxford, U.K.

Summary

The problems confronting patients with epilepsy, their families, and the surgeons wishing to help such patients, are discussed. It is important for physicians in other specialities to realise that epilepsy surgery is not nowadays complex, difficult, painful or uncertain; furthermore such operations are based on finding and removing focal lesions rather than "epileptogenic cortex" and the result in terms of integration of the patient into society is much improved if such intervention is performed while the patient is young, with time to gain academic and social skills after the operation.

The selection of patients suitable for operation is discussed as well as methods of determining which hemisphere is dominant for speech and whether or not the focal lesion involves language centres.

The majority of patients with drug resistant epilepsy suitable for operation have abnormalities in one temporal lobe. The pathological lesion is described and the advantages and disadvantages of various operations for temporal lobe epilepsy discussed. Extra-temporal cortical resection in the dominant hemisphere is also considered, particularly with reference to the preservation of language function.

It is important that neurosurgeons realise that MRI and CT scanning have transformed epilepsy surgery from being a rather nebulous, time consuming art, to being for the majority of patients, a clear cut, straight forward procedure firmly based on "Oslerian" pathological principles. Far too few patients are being offered an operation (which renders 60–70% seizure free); neurosurgeons should respond to this challenge.

Keywords: Epilepsy; surgery; language function, indications; results.

Introduction

Hippocrates in his monograph on the "sacred disease" established that epilepsy arose from the brain. Galen, and his teacher Pelops, decided that the auras of seizures were vapours of humours travelling from the peripheral parts of the body to the brain so as to cause the seizures. In the seventeenth century Charles Le Pois and Thomas Willis are credited with establishing that the auras and the epilepsy both arise from the brain. Thomas Willis who also described the arterial *circle (or polygon) of Willis, lived in Oxford in a house* which is still standing (Fig. 1).

On July 13th 1886 Victor Horsley[7] first operated for epilepsy. His patient was twenty-four years of age. At the age of five while working as a stable boy (a commentary in those times) a carriage shaft fell on his head producing a compound penetrating fracture in the right frontal area. At the age of 13 he was kicked by a horse in the same spot and three months later developed epilepsy with a rectal aura and jerking of the right hand. Horsley performed a craniotomy and excised the scar finding a fragment of bone within the brain. The patient made a good recovery and in 1909 Horsley reported him to be in "robust health". Horsley was a remarkable man. He was colour-blind, perfectly ambidextrous and fluent in French and German. He was a man of remarkably broad social interests. Yet ironically his only and beloved son developed epilepsy and Horsley himself was required to operate upon his own child. "What demon" wrote Osler "drove a man of this type into the muddy pool of politics?" Horsley suddenly retired at the age of 49. Perhaps the answer lies, as Dr David Taylor[15] suggests, in his son's epilepsy. "How could he have borne to be visited through his own son, with what he had laboured so fiercely to conquer in his patients".

Epilepsy is a most trying disorder for the patient to bear. The crux of this burden is the reaction of society to that disease. But the fact that Society imposes this burden on the sufferer does not diminish the difficulties. When one cures a patient of epilepsy one not only cures the patient but cures the family as well. Parents can go out together again; brothers and sisters can bring home friends for the first time, while the patient no longer seeks refuge from life. So often one sees children passing through their teenage years becoming recluses and one of the many pleas I shall be giving in this contribution, is the need to operate on children rather

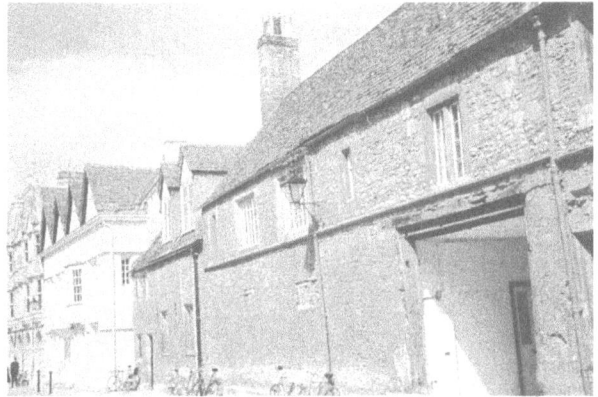

Fig. 1. Thomas Willis' House, still standing in Merton Street, Oxford

than on adults, so that there is time to rehabilitate them socially and academically. The best results in terms of reintegration into society undoubtedly occur when the epilepsy is cured in youth rather than adult life. In the past the person with epilepsy, especially epilepsy arising from the temporal lobe, was branded as being possessed by the devil, or by the occult and many in the past were subjected to being burnt to death. Today society is less cruel, but people's reactions are determined so much by ignorance, fear and indeed, fear of fear.

There is another problem concerning epilepsy and this problem is not society's ignorance, but the ignorance of the medical profession. After Horsley, Penfield and Foerster[6] successfully operated on patients with epilepsy following low velocity penetrating injuries to the brain. The Montreal School pioneered epilepsy surgery particularly using the EEG and Electrocorticography to guide the extent of excision. The concept arose that epilepsy surgery required finding and removing "epileptogenic cortex". The pre-operative investigations became lengthy and complex; the operation – usually under local anaesthesia – was arduous for the patient and the surgeon and the results were uncertain. Some colleagues felt that it was illogical to substitute epileptogenic cortex by a surgical scar. Thus the surgery of epilepsy became and has to some extent remained a rarified form of surgery confined to a few centres in the world. Indeed I believe I am right in saying there is no epilepsy surgery performed in Japan. Doctors, indeed neurologists, paediatricians and even many neurosurgeons regard this surgery as too complicated to be considered for patients. The consequence of this attitude is that there are many patients with epilepsy who could be cured of their disease yet have not been properly assessed with a view to operation.

I wish to change this attitude. Epilepsy surgery is, in the majority of patients, a straight-forward procedure with good results in properly selected patients. The concept of "epileptogenic cortex" must go. The tragedy of the early years of the Montreal School is that there was no adequate pathological examination of the specimens, for the brain was sucked away until the spikes disappeared and such specimens that were obtained were biopsies. This technique is somewhat irreverently called "spike chasing". This too must go because we know that persistence of spikes after excision does not indicate the result of surgery. The proper approach to epilepsy surgery should be to find and remove focal pathology. The concept of occult focal pathology must now replace the concept of "epileptogenic cortex" and thus allow surgery to return to the well tried, clearly understood Oslerian concept of the pathological basis of disease and its treatment. I must emphasize that good results follow when focal pathology is found and removed, but when no lesion is found in the specimen then the results are much less certain. Furthermore operations that do not involve excising tissue have not withstood the test of time. There have been many different procedures tried in the past; indeed they constitute an index of the desperation and bravery of the patient and the surgeon alike.

I will illustrate my approach by describing a patient called Jeremy. I saw him in 1974 at the age of 16. He lived in the North Of England and started having psychomotor epilepsy at the age of 11. This consisted of episodes in which he would "switch off" his colour changed to grey or purple, but he would continue to stand or walk. He might rub his hands on a table or nearby object in a repetitive manner. In addition he had several grand mal attacks and on average was having two to three attacks per day despite large doses of anti-convulsants. His behaviour deteriorated; he was violent, threatening his family and breaking furniture.

He was referred to London for consideration of an operation. The EEG showed bilateral independent spike activity at both sphenoidal leads and so he was turned down for any operation (Fig. 2). I saw him for a further opinion and noted a speck of calcification in the right temporal lobe and the air encephalogram showed a slightly dilated temporal horn. I felt that a focal lesion had been demonstrated and that therefore the EEG should be ignored.

In March 1974 I performed a right 6 cm *en bloc* temporal lobectomy and found 4 cm from the temporal pole, a hard, purple mass some 2 cm in diameter (Fig. 3). This was reported as an oligodendroglioma. Post-operatively his epilepsy stopped immediately and of great interest, the post-operative EEG showed cessation of abnormal activity in the contralateral temporal lobe. His behaviour became normal. Subsequently he went to University, got married and now leads a normal life. The point I wish to emphasize is the importance of finding and removing any focal lesion, rather than removing epileptogenic cortex. Thus, here is a patient with apparently independent spike activity from both sphenoidal leads yet with just a focal lesion in one temporal lobe.

There is a further point I must make. There is a

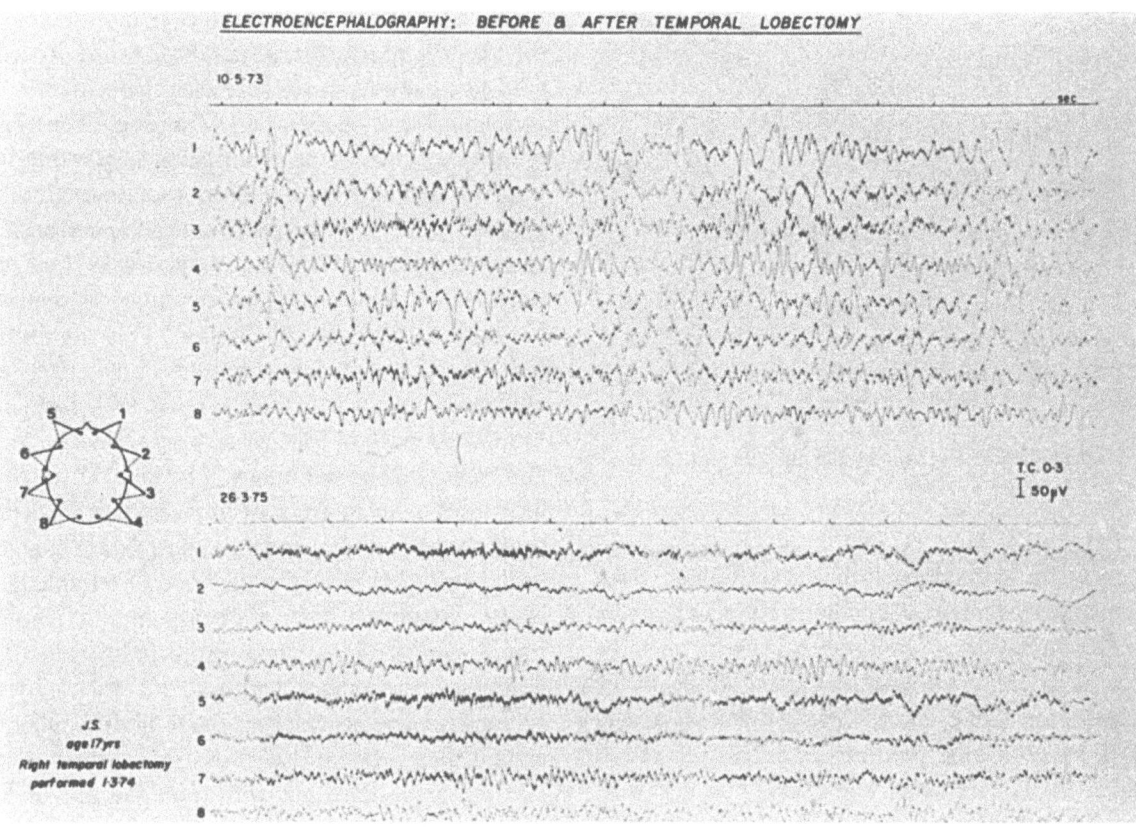

Fig. 2. *EEG* traces to show (pre-operatively) bilateral independent spikes from the temporal lobes which were no longer seen post-operatively after removal of a right temporal, two centimetre diameter, indolent glioma

regrettable tendency to make the pre-operative investigations of these patients extremely complex. Neurophysiological investigations must include the EEG, particularly with the patient asleep. Sphenoidal leads are also essential if there is a possibility of epilepsy arising from the temporal lobe. However, some colleagues are now advocating implanting electrodes and

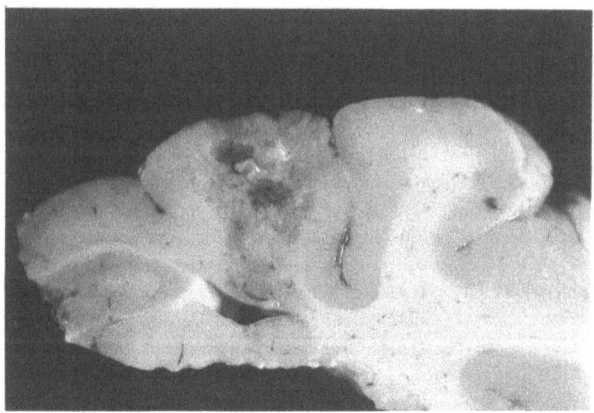

Fig. 3. Histological appearances of the two centimetre indolent oligodendroglioma in the right temporal lobe causing bi-temporal independent spikes

long term video monitoring. Foramen ovale electrodes are being more frequently inserted. These investigations require a lengthy period of time in hospital, sometimes quite considerable pain and discomfort for the patient, as well as requiring on occasions, operative placement of subdural electrodes and even implantation of electrodes into the brain substance, which itself raises questions about the possibility of exacerbating the epileptic process.

Engel[4] in the USA estimates that between one hundred thousand and two hundred fifty thousand patients might benefit from epilepsy surgery. Yet fewer than three hundred such operations are performed each year in the USA. Of patients suitable for epilepsy surgery 80% do *not* require complex, painful, dangerous and lengthy pre-operative investigations. The 20% that do, probably obtain less good results from operation as the criteria for intervention are obviously less clear-cut in this group. I would suggest we concentrate our restricted resources on those patients who are obvious candidates for operation. The results will be better, more patients will be treated and of particular importance, referring neurologists, paediatricians and other doctors, will become more confident about referring patients to us.

Indications for Epilepsy Surgery

The indication for an operation is essentially the presence of an occult focal lesion causing epilepsy, which itself is refractory to medical treatment and that the focal lesion can be removed without harm to the patient[12]. I shall consider the question of speech function later. Some authors have stated that the patient should be having more than a certain number of fits per month and that the IQ should be greater than a particular figure. With respect I disagree. Even one fit per month, may be incapacitating. Why should a low IQ deny a person a chance of being rid of another disability? Another important factor is behaviour. Why some epileptic children develop behaviour problems is not known. However, it is my experience that if one stops the epilepsy the behaviour returns to normal. This is often an important factor to be taken into consideration particularly in the group of hemiplegic children under consideration for hemispherectomy.

What methods therefore do we have to determine if there is any focal lesion? There are four ways;

1. The History

The importance of a careful history is too often ignored. If the epilepsy always starts in the same way, or with the same aura, then this is very suggestive of a local origin for the epilepsy. It does not matter how the seizure develops; it may develop in different ways and severity, but if it always commences in the same way,

then the clinician should be alerted to the possibility of an underlying focal pathological lesion.

2. CT Scan

Temporal lobectomy is the most common operation for epilepsy and about 70% of all such operations for epilepsy have been performed on the temporal lobe. Of course standard CT scanning shows high and low density lesions, especially calcification, and it is an essential investigation. But the importance of temporal orientated CT scanning cannot be over-emphasized (Fig. 4). This orientation allows the shape and size of the temporal lobes and horns to be accurately assessed. Intrathecal contrast is also helpful to delineate the medial aspect of the temporal lobes (Fig. 5). Not infrequently temporal lobe pathology is missed because of failure to carry out temporal orientated CT scans.

3. MRI

MRI is the best method for delineating the shape and size of the temporal lobe as well as showing the pathology within (Fig. 6). Mesial temporal, or Ammon's Horn sclerosis, will in future be diagnosed with more sophisticated MRI. The disadvantage of MRI is that it does not show calcification and thus the two methods of imaging are complimentary. Measuring the volume of the hippocampus is becoming an important and in-

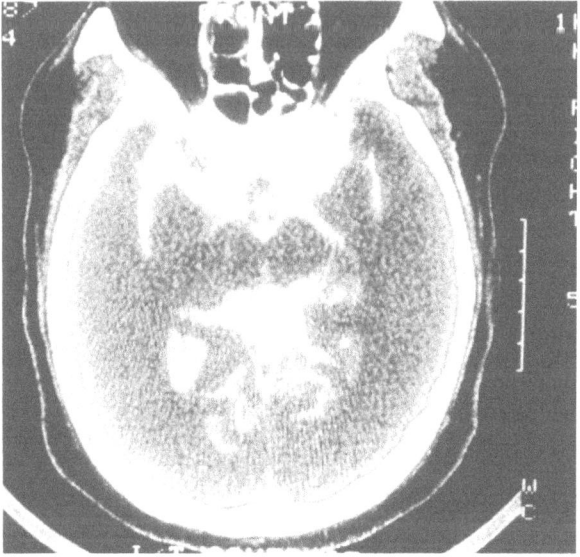

Fig. 5. Intrathecal contrast with temporal orientated CT scanning delineates the medial aspect of the temporal lobes particularly well; Coronal scanning with the intrathecal contrast also demonstrates clearly the temporal lobe atrophy

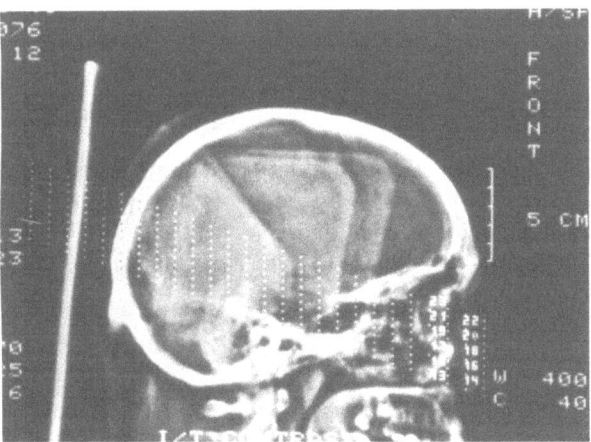

Fig. 4. Temporal orientated CT scanning is essential for imaging the temporal lobe

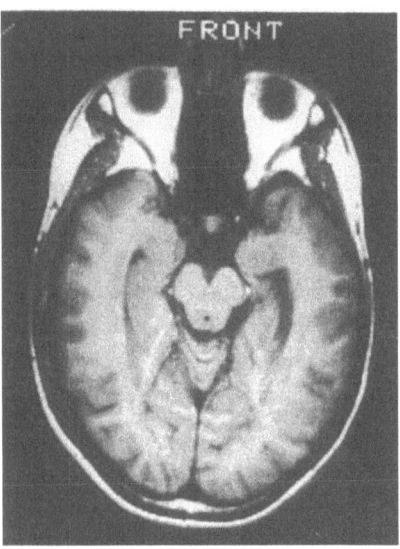

Fig. 6. MRI is the best method to delineate the shape and size of the temporal lobe as well as showing pathology within. This MRI shows atrophy of the left temporal lobe and hippocampus with enlargement of the temporal horn

expensive method of assessing temporal lobe epilepsy patients.

4. EEG

Although I have cautioned against excessive reliance on the EEG it still has, of course, an important place in the investigation of these patients. The EEG and the clinical history are the only ways of determining whether or not the abnormalities seen on imaging are in fact causing the epilepsy. Essentially, spikes represent epileptic activity, and slow waves pathology. The importance of inducing sleep to enhance spike activity must be emphasised. I have already made the point that spikes may arise from a focal lesion in the opposite hemisphere.

Epilepsy arising outside the temporal lobe does require pre-operative electrocorticography to locate the pathology, especially if imaging fails to show any abnormality.

These therefore are the four ways of determining focal pathology.

Epilepsy Surgery in the Speech Area

It is now necessary to consider the more specific question of epilepsy operations in the speech area. The ability to speak is fundamental and most people would consider its loss too high a price for abolishing epilepsy. The effects of operating on the dominant temporal lobe

are of course not only aphasia or dysphasia but also difficulty in reading, writing, spelling and calculating. There is also a more subtle difficulty of remembering verbal information or verbal memory as the psychologists refer to it. Dr. and Mrs. Oxbury have studied this aspect of the Oxford series of temporal lobectomy patients[12]. Verbal memory is reduced after temporal lobectomy especially in the group with small indolent gliomas or hamartomas. There is less deterioration in patients with Ammon's Horn sclerosis, because perhaps the pre-existing damage to the hippocampus and amygdala has already caused verbal memory impairment and the additional surgical insult is of less consequence.

Unfortunately there is little agreement between the various psychologists studying these patients. Different psychologists use different tests and their task is not helped by the variation in operative technique from surgeon to surgeon when performing a temporal lobectomy. Some surgeons remove just neocortex leaving the amygdala and hippocampus. Others remove the amygdala, hippocampus and parahippocampus, but spare the neocortex, while yet others do an *en bloc* removal of both neocortex and hippocampus, but taking varying lengths of the hippocampus. Psychologists applying their various tests to these various groups find, it seems, verbal memory loss in all groups, with poor correlation with the extent of hippocampal removal. The only certain fact is that bilateral hippocampal removal causes severe, indeed catastrophic memory loss. Removal of the dominant temporal lobe will cause verbal memory loss and probably the greater the amount of normal tissue removed, the greater the extent of verbal memory loss. There is a need for more standardized tests and more tests which reflect everyday tasks carried out in life, rather than the artificial environment of the psychologists laboratory.

The Determination of the Dominant Hemisphere

The surgeon needs to know which hemisphere is dominant for speech, especially when the patient is left-handed when the dominance may be either left or right or distributed between the two hemispheres. It is rare for a right-handed person to be right hemisphere dominant, but I have had a such a patient. Ojemann[10] states that one per cent of right handed patients have language dominance in the right hemisphere and so one must be careful not to assume that right-handed patients are invariably left hemisphere dominant for speech.

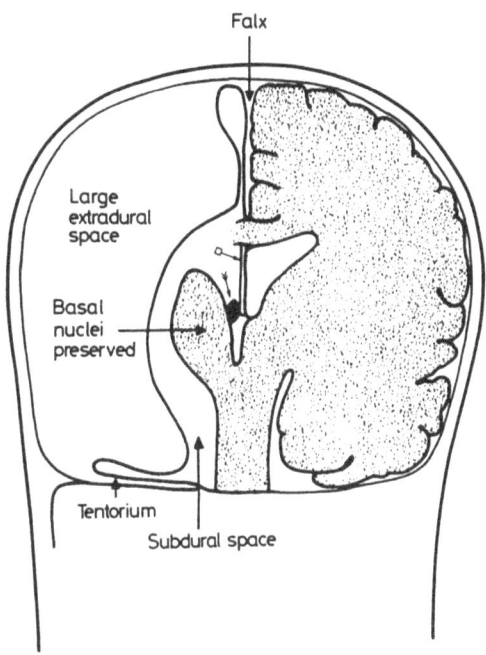

Fig. 7. Oxford modification of the hemispherectomy operation to prevent delayed complications

There may be some clinical indication of the dominance; if the seizure is associated with speech arrest and transient post-ictal dysphasia, then clearly the focus is in the dominant hemisphere. Repetitive speech during a seizure indicates an origin in the non-dominant hemisphere.

Absolute confirmation is obtained by the Wada test which entails anaesthetizing each hemisphere by injecting Amytal into either carotid artery The psychologists then test two functions, speech and memory. Memory is tested to exclude the total amnesic syndrome which occurs after unilateral temporal lobectomy if the remaining hippocampus is damaged or non-functioning. Unfortunately this test cannot be administered in children under the age of twelve. In the group of hemiplegic children with severe epilepsy and behaviour disorder, being considered for hemispherectomy, speech impairment need not be a cause of concern to the surgeon. The brain shows remarkable plasticity so that damage to the dominant hemisphere up to the age of five years will allow the transfer of speech to the unaffected side, although this transfer occurs more gradually the older the child. Hemispherectomy is still the best operation for epilepsy; we in Oxford have modified the standard technique (Fig. 7) and have used this modification since 1980 without the delayed bleeding complications that caused this operation to be abandoned in the late 1960s[2]. This modification has

two objectives, the first to prevent blood seeping into the ventricular system by plugging the Foramen of Munro and secondly to obliterate the large operative subdural cavity by creating an extradural space[1].

The *exact sites of the speech areas in the dominant hemisphere* continues to attract debate. Penfield and Jasper[13] describe "stimulatory arrest" of speech. This technique depends on applying a stimulating electrode to the speech area in patients undergoing craniotomy under local anaesthesia. Penfield found that by avoiding excision of these areas of stimulatory arrest of speech, post-operative aphasia could be prevented. It shoud be noted that this technique of stimulating by way of electrodes produces speech arrest, although stimulation in the same manner in the region of the motor or sensory cortex produces movement or sensation rather than cessation of these functions.

Penfield and Jasper[13], and later Penfield and Roberts[14] concluded that there were four areas of cortex devoted to speech in the dominant hemisphere. These are the inferior frontal or Broca's area; the second and third areas are respectively the inferior parietal and posterior temporal regions and these are known jointly as Wernicke's speech area. The fourth area is the superior frontal area adjacent to the falx just in front of the leg area of the motor cortex near the supplementary motor area. All these areas produce speech arrest with electrical stimulation but the fourth or last area can be excised without persistent speech deficit although temporary speech disturbance, even mutism, may occur.

Ojemann[11] has given us a careful assessment of cortical language localization. He is right to use the term "cortical" because there is increasing evidence of aphasia developing after sub-cortical damage especially in the thalamic area where the pulvinar seems particularly important for speech. Stimulation or damage to the pulvinar causes anomia or difficulty in naming objects and I know of one patient who became aphasic after a temporal lobectomy performed for epilepsy, as a result of damage to the thalamo-geniculate branches of the posterior cerebral artery, which, of course, winds around the brain stem particularly in the region of the pulvinar of the thalamus. Brodal[3] summarises the evidence for subcortical damage causing aphasia and also makes the important point that although we speak of speech centres, this is too crude an anatomical concept for such a complex function as speech. Nevertheless as surgeons we need this simplistic approach to the speech function of our patients.

George Ojemann has spent many years studying

speech localization during epilepsy surgery and his must be the most authoritative opinion on this subject. This recent publication records the results of studying 117 patients[11]. He too assesses the effect of cortical stimulation on the patient's ability to name objects. He makes several important points.

The "language centres" are highly localised. In two-thirds of his patients there are two discrete areas for language, each measuring between one and two square centimetres. One quarter of the patients had three or more such areas. Usually a patient has one language area in the inferior frontal or Broca's area and one or two language centres in the inferior parietal or posterior superior temporal gyrus, in other words, Wernicke's area. However the total area for language is far smaller than the traditional view and is about a quarter of the area delineated by Penfield and Roberts. However these areas are subject to great individual variability of size and position. Despite this each area in the individual is remarkably well defined. That is to say there is only occasionally a gradation of language function as one moves away from the site of the stimulatory anomia. Ojemann argues that sites of evoked naming errors do represent sites of essential language function that cannot be excised without language impairment. His diagram (Fig. 8) summarises the variable and widespread sites of simulatory anomia and he asserts that anatomical localization of speech cannot be relied upon. Indeed in some patients the classical Broca's area is uninvolved with language.

Yet with all techniques there are difficulties even with so carefully an applied technique such as Ojemann's. It is indeed curious that one uses stimulation to inhibit speech. This suggests that the language centres found by this technique are not speech centres but more precisely, centers when stimulated actually inhibit the ability to name objects. Ojemann in fact describes cases in which speech is maintained but naming ability falters. Furthermore preservation of these areas does not necessarily preserve all language function such as reading or indeed verbal memory. There is evidence that the fusiform gyrus on the inferior aspect of the temporal lobe may be important for speech and this cannot of course be assessed by stimulation. Indeed Ojemann has found language centres in such widespread areas, that the surgeon may be forgiven for being perplexed. Should a localised lesion causing epilepsy far removed from the traditional speech areas *not* be removed, should stimulation reveal impaired naming ability in such an area? Furthermore the effects of a lesion in the cortex must be different from that of stimulation, for in the former situation some functional adaptation can occur which obviously cannot operate during stimulation. The technique is difficult, time-consuming and usually requires the craniotomy to be performed under local anaesthesia, and I have argued already for the desirability of operating on young people rather than adults which must restrict the use of this technique at least for the group of patients I see.

Ojemann advises that there should be at least a two centimetre margin of cortex preserved around the stimulatory language centres during cortical resection. I myself carry out an *en bloc* six centimetre temporal lobectomy, but sparing the posterior half of the superior temporal gyrus on the dominant side. The only patient who was dysphasic post-operatively had a post-operative clot; the *en bloc* temporal lobectomy has not itself caused any significant dysphasia (at most an impairment of speech fluency) and this suggests to me that the prolonged stressful procedure under local anaesthesia is necessary if speech centres are to be determined for each individual, may not in fact be necessary, especially if a focal lesion is considered the essential lesion to remove rather than epileptogenic cortex. Indeed in non temporal lobe epilepsy, a focal lesion even in Broca's or Wernicke's areas may be excised without undue risk of speech impairment if none existed pre-operatively.

Finally perhaps it is not inappropriate in our Academy to point out that "language" differs between nations and perhaps language based on morphograms differs in cortical localization from syllabogram

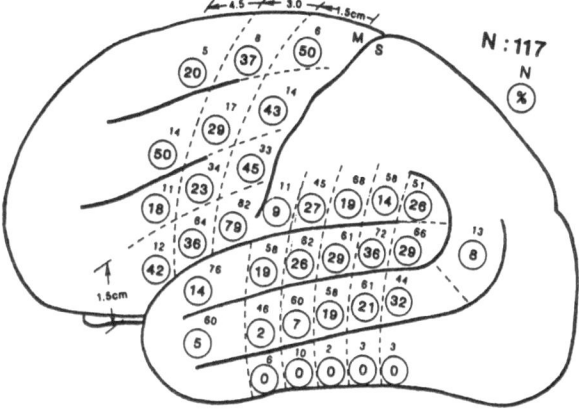

Fig. 8. Diagram by George Ojemann summarising his data on the localization of language centres in 117 patients. The cortex is divided into zones identified by dashed lines. Upper number in each zone is the number of patients with a site in that zone; lower number in circle is the percentage of those patients with significant naming errors in that zone. M and S indicate motor (*M*) or sensory (*S*) Cortex

language. I refer to the paper of Yokata *et al.* describing pure agraphia to kanji yet preservation of Kana[18].

The Surgery of Epilepsy

I now turn to the operative aspects; the most common cause for drug resistant epilepsy is that arising from the temporal lobes and temporal lobectomy accounts for 70% of all operations performed worldwide for epilepsy. Drug resistance should not be assumed unless there are unacceptably frequent seizures despite maximum tolerable doses of at least three different drugs taken singly or in combination[12].

There are two common pathologies in the temporal lobe. The first is *Ammon's horn (or mesial temporal) sclerosis*. This is loss of neurones in the hippocampus with gliosis. The cause is a prolonged (i.e. longer than thirty minutes) febrile convulsion in a young person, that is under four years of age. It seems that the amygdala and hippocampus of the young immature brain are particularly sensitive to prolonged convulsions producing a self destructive process or "consumptive" anoxia. It is not known why this process is predominantly unilateral. Many of these children develop a transient contralateral hemiplegia as well and I personally can see a gradation from this to the group of children who at around the age of two develop a febrile illness associated with severe epilepsy which culminates in infantile hemiplegia and drug resistant epilepsy; these children are those that come to hemispherectomy, but even so, it is quite unknown why the illness is so profoundly unilateral.

A few years after the prolonged febrile convulsion, usually at around the age of five or six, these children start to develop psychomotor epilepsy. Three-quarters have an aura, typically an epigastric sensation rising up to the throat. The patient experiences psychical features, such as fear, memory flashbacks or hallucinations, while an observer sees motor phenomena typically swallowing, lip smacking or repetitive limb movements. On the dominant side the patient may be dysphasic for a while after the seizure.

The second most common lesion is an *indolent glioma*; these are probably hamartomas of astrocytes or oligodendroglia; they are frequently calcified. Why they predominate in the temporal lobes is not known. Nor do we know if they have a propensity to turn malignant. The curious fact is that although such lesions must have been present all that patient's life, the epilepsy typically does not start until the age of eight or nine. It is as if the brain requires a certain

En Bloc Temporal Lobectomy - Falconer

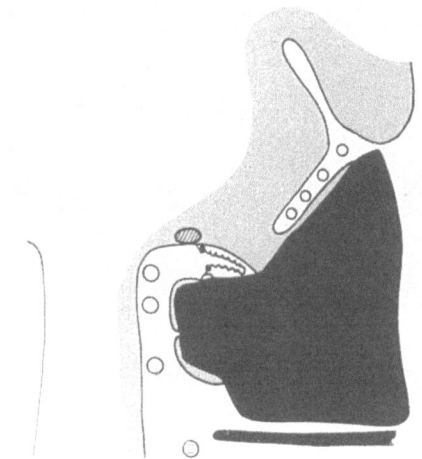

Fig. 9. Diagram showing the *en bloc* temporal lobectomy pioneered by Murray Falconer. The preservation of pia-arachnoid against the brain stem and medial to the free edge of the tentorium is particularly important

degree of maturation before psychomotor epilepsy can commence.

In my series 90% of the patient have one or other of these two pathological lesions. Two-thirds have Mesial temporal sclerosis and one-third glial hamartomas. The history must not only explore the consistency of the epileptic attack but also the past history of prolonged febrile convulsion or any transient hemiplegia following such an event.

Although I have stressed the importance of removing a focal lesion, I have to add that the results of operation for temporal lobe epilepsy are better if the amygdala and hippocampus are also removed with the specific lesion. It seems that the epileptic process is channelled through these structures. I carry out two procedures for drug-resistant epilepsy arising from the dominant temporal lobe. The first is an "*en bloc*" temporal lobectomy pioneered by the late Murray Falconer[5] (Fig. 9). This extends six centimetres behind the temporal pole and spares the posterior part of the superior temporal gyrus. This procedure has the advantage of removing any widespread lesion within the temporal lobe and at the same time producing a good specimen for pathological examination. It is a well-tested procedure. The disadvantage is that of an inevitable upper quadrantic visual field loss, which in ten per cent of patients extends to an hemianopic loss, presumably due to individual variations in Myer's loop of the optic radiation.

An important point in the technique of this operation

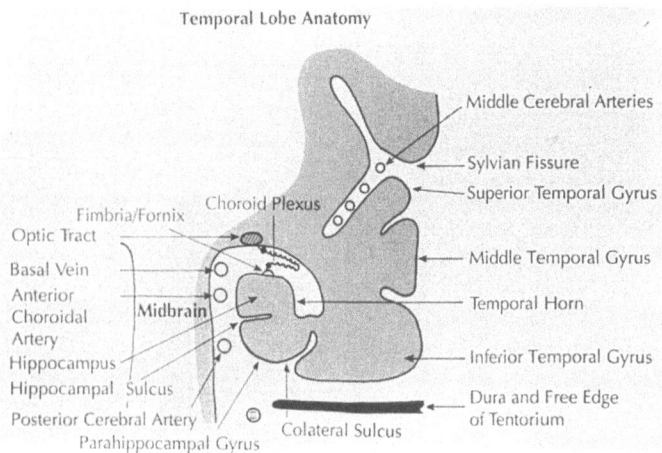

Fig. 10. Diagram to show the vessels and other structures that should be preserved during operations on the temporal lobe

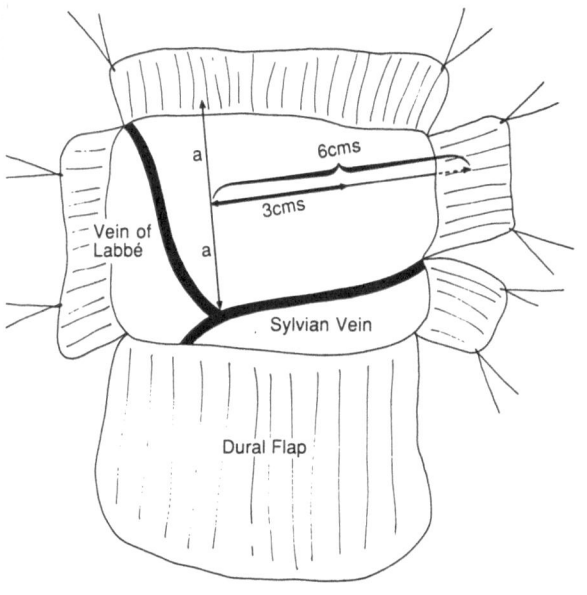

Temporal Horn Found at 4.0 cms

Fig. 12. Incision used for the Oxford microsurgical modification of Neimyer's amygdalo-hippocampectomy

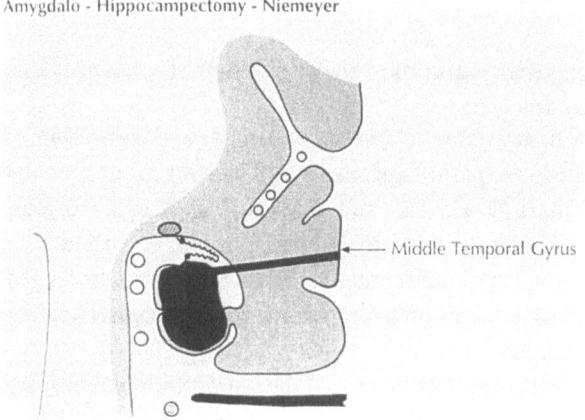

Fig. 11. Selective amygdalo-hippocampectomy after Neimyer. Diagram to show the approach and structures removed

is to preserve the the pia-archnoid overlying the midbrain and associated vessels (Fig. 10).

The risk of dysphasia using this approach is very small. Only one patient, as I have mentioned, has had temporary aphasia. Transient mild dysphasia may last for a few weeks. I have had one patient who has had a transient hemiplegia following this procedure because of a post-operative clot.

I have already referred to verbal memory loss and, if anything, this is more disabling than dysphasia. It is necessary to discuss this disability with patients and their relatives, especially if the patient is involved in academic work.

The second procedure is that of *amygdalo-hippocampectomy*. This operation spares the neocortex of the temporal lobe but removes the hippocampus, amygdala and parahippocampal gyrus. This operation is done in two ways. The transcortical approach, by way of an incision in the middle temporal gyrus was first described by Neimyer in 1958[9] (Fig. 11). Since 1989 we have been using a microsurgical procedure utilising this approach (Fig. 12). In 1982 Yaşargil described a selective amygdalo-hippocampectomy using a pterional approach (Fig. 13). There are advantages and disadvantages for this selective operation and indeed for the two different approaches. The selective operation is undoubtedly less upsetting for the patient. There is less post-operative morbidity, perhaps because less dura is exposed. It is hoped there is less verbal memory impairment and a smaller chance

Amygdalo - Hippocampectomy - Yasargil

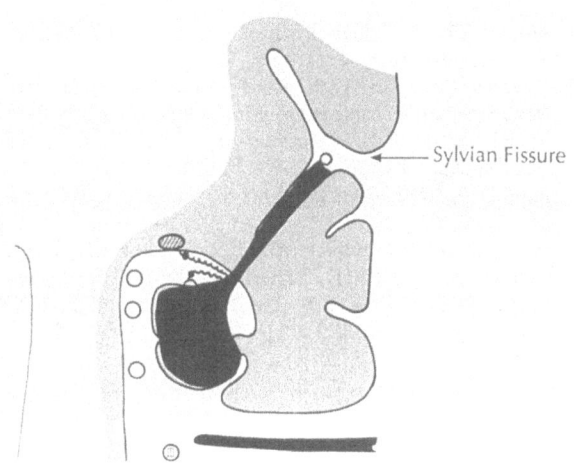

Sylvian Fissure

Fig. 13. Diagram to show Yaşargil's pterional selective amygdalo-hippocampectomy. The advantages and disadvantages of these procedures are discussed in the text

of a visual field defect. Clearly the risk of dysphasia must be smaller after this procedure, but I have already made the point that this is very small after *en bloc* lobectomy sparing the posterior part of the superior temporal gyrus. However the selective operation is unsuitable for a diffuse lesion in the temporal lobe, though obviously it is especially indicated for those patients with conditions such as mesial temporal sclerosis or an indolent glioma confined to the region of the amygdala or hippocampus.

The advantage of Yaşargil's approach is that neocortex is spared and theoretically there should be no visual field defect. The disadvantage of this approach is the limited exposure and the inability to obtain a good specimen for pathological study, as well as the possibility of damage to the middle cerebral, anterior choroidal and posterior cerebral arterises as well as the optic tract. The advantage of the transcortical approach is that the exposure is better, and *en bloc* removal of the amygdala, hippocampus and parahippocampal gyrus can be achieved; if necessary one has the flexibility to perform a lobectomy or larger excision.

Although Yaşargil's results are comparable to *en bloc* temporal lobectomy, as far as relief of epilepsy is concerned, we do not yet know if his selective approach produces less verbal memory deficit. The initial reports from Zurich suggested that this was so, but later reports, and reports from other units using Yaşargil's approach, have in fact reported a significant number of patients with significant verbal memory deficits. I have already referred to the difficulty in assessing

verbal memory deficits, not only because of the differing methods of testing used by psychologists, but also the varying amounts of tissues removed by surgeons from different parts of the temporal lobe. We still do not know whether it is the amygdala, hippocampus or indeed parahippocampal gyrus, let alone the neocortex that is responsible for verbal memory. Perhaps all four structures subserve verbal memory and if this is the case any operation removing these structures will produce a deficit.

In Oxford we feel that the *en bloc* temporal lobectomy produces better results in terms of seizure control than the selective operation. We therefore use the *en bloc* temporal lobectomy for non-dominant temporal lobe epilepsy or for dominant temporal lobe epilepsy when the lesion extends beyond the amygdala and hippocampus. We use the transcortical selective amygdalo-hippocampectomy for dominant temporal lobe epilepsy if the lesion is confined to the amygdala, hippocampus or parahippocampal gyrus.

Less commonly epilepsy arises in other parts of the dominant hemisphere and speech may be involved in the manifestation of the epilepsy or be at risk from operations for epilepsy arising in these areas. The clinician should be alerted to the risk if speech arrest occurs during the seizure, or if there is transient dysphasia in the post-ictal period. Furthermore continuous subclinical seizure activity itself may cause profound, long-standing speech disturbance, and I have had one patient who demonstrated this. Thus aphasia maybe a functional aphasia due to epileptic discharges causing speech arrest, rather than a structural aphasia from the presence of the lesion in the speech area.

It is my view that a focal lesion arising in the language area producing epilepsy can be removed without causing unacceptable aphasia. I say this because if the patient is able to talk, then this lesion must have allowed adaption of normal language mechanisms to have occurred. Thus such a lesion can be removed without deficit. But the removal must be precisely that of the lesion and one is not able to remove surrounding cortex on the basis that it may be epileptogenic. Nor is one allowed to excise "epileptogenic cortex" which does not contain a pathological lesion. Such operation does require electrocorticography but in my view the use of local anaesthesia and speech mapping is not a practical proposition, because the patients referred for this type of operation, are children.

Morrell, Whisler and Bleck[8] have recently described

a procedure of *multiple sub-pial transection in patients with epilepsy arising in eloquent areas.* Their approach is remove the focal lesion and then perform sub-pial transection on adjacent "epileptogenic cortex". Of the twenty patients all but two had a structural lesion and so it is difficult to know if their figure of fifty five per cent complete control of seizures is due to the removal of the structural lesion or the undermining of the adjacent so-called epileptogenic cortex. No patients suffered a clinically significant deficit and this paper is quoted to highlight the fact that the surgeon can indeed remove structural lesions in eloquent areas of the brain without serious deficit.

In summary, operations for epilepsy are performed less than they should be. Many patients suffering epilepsy, or to use Professor David Taylor's term, suffering "a passport to prejudice" could be rid of their epilepsy, if only doctors considered the possibility of operation. We neurosurgeons must emphasize to our colleagues that this procedure is based on secure pathological principles. Although of course neurophysiology is still of great importance, the development of sophisticated imaging methods has allowed subtle epileptogenic lesions to be identified. It is to *this* that surgeons must direct their attention rather than adjacent, so-called, epileptogenic cortex. The presence of such a lesion in the dominant temporal lobe may be treated by *en bloc* temporal lobectomy or selective amygdalo-hippocam-pectomy depending on its actual extent. Lesions else-where in the speech area may be removed by micro neurosurgical techniques without serious language deficits.

In conclusion, sophisticated imaging has transformed the operative treatment of epilepsy and we as neurosurgeons must accept this challenge.

Acknowledgements

It is a pleasure to thank Dr. and Mrs. Oxbury for their help in this work. I also thank the Editors of the Journals of Neurosurgery and Neurology, Neurosurgery and Psychiatry for their permission to reproduce Figs. 8 and 7.

References

1. Adams CBT (1983) Hemispherectomy, a modification. J Neurol Neurosurg Psychiatry 46: 617–619
2. Beardworth ED, Adams CBT (1988) Modified hemispherectomy for epilepsy: early results in ten cases. Br J Neurosurg 2: 73–84
3. Brodal A (1981) Neurological anatomy in relation to clinical medicine, 2nd Ed. Oxford Medical Publications
4. Engel J (1987) Surgical treatment of the epilepsies. Raven Press, New York
5. Falconer MA (1971) Operative surgery. In: Rob C, Smith H. (eds) Neurosurgery, 2nd Ed. Butterworths, London, pp 142–149
6. Foerster O, Penfield W (1930) The structural basis of traumatic epilepsy and results of radical operation. Brain 54: 99–120
7. Horsley V (1886) Brain surgery. Br Med J 1: 670–675
8. Morrell F, Whisler WW, Bleck TP (1989) Multiple subpial transection: a new approach to the Surgical treatment of focal epilepsy. J Neurosurg 70: 231–239
9. Neimyer P (1958) The transventicular amygdalo-hippocampectomy in temporal lobe epilepsy. In: Baldwin R., Maitland H. et al. (eds) Temporal lobe epilepsy. Charles C Thomas, Springfield, pp 461–482
10. Ojemann GA (1987) Intraoperative functional mapping at the University of Seattle. In: Engel J (ed) Surgical treatment of the epilepsies. Raven Press, New York
11. Ojemann GA, Ojemann J, Lettich E, Berger M (1989) Cortical language localization in left dominant hemisphere. J Neurosurg 71: 316–326
12. Oxbury JM, Adams CBT (1989) Neurosurgery for epilepsy. Br J Hosp Med 41: 372–378
13. Penfield W, Jasper H (1954) Epilepsy and the functional anatomy of the human brain. Little, Brown, Boston
14. Penfield W, Roberts L (1959) Speech and brain mechanisms. Princeton University Press, New Jersey
15. Taylor DC (1987) One hundred years of epilepsy surgery: Sir Victor Horsley's contribution. In: Engel J (ed) Surgical treatment of the epilepsies. Raven Press, New York, pp 7–11
16. Wieser HG, Yaşargil MG (1982) Selective amygdalo-hippocampectomy as a surgical treatment of mesiobasal limbic epilepsy. Surg Neurol 17: 445–457
17. Yaşargil MG, Teddy PJ, Roth P (1985) Selective amygdalo-hippocampectomy, operative anatomy and surgical techniques. In: Symon L et al (eds) Advances and technical standards in neurosurgery, Vol 12. Springer, Berlin Heidelberg New York Tokyo
18. Yokota T, Ishial S, Furukawa T, Tsukagoshi H (1990) Pure Agraphia of Kanji due to thrombosis of the labbé vein. J Neurol Neurosurg Psychiatry 53: 335–338

Correspondence: C.B.T. Adams, M. Chir FRCS, Department of Neurosurgery, Radcliffe Infirmary, Oxford OX2 6HE UK.

Acta Neurochirurgica (1993) [Suppl] 56: 83–84

Lateralisation of Speech Centre in Left-Handedness Due to Cerebral and Extracerebral Lesions

K. Srinivasan

Department of Neurology and Neurosurgery, Medical College Madurai, India

Summary

This report is based on a study of a small sample of five patients who were initially right-handed and became left-handed due to loss of function in the right arm after extracerebral causes such as polio or injury. Carotid amytal tests in these patients showed that all of them still had the speech centre in the left hemisphere. As expected, lateralised neuropsychological brain function tests showed no significant differences between right and left brain.

In infantile right hemiplegia due to atrophic left brain lesions, the speech centre had shifted to right side in 10 out of 15 patients. Neuropsychological tests showed sparing and protection of dominant left brain functions.

Keywords: Lefthandness; speech centre; lateralization.

Introduction

The left hemisphere is considered dominant because of the location of the speech centre. In most of the right-handed or left-handed persons, symbolic and propositional expressive speech seems to be exclusively located in the left hemisphere whereas a number of other higher cerebral or mental functions fall within the scope of either hemisphere. With a left hemisphere lesion or excision in early life, the right brain takes over language functions and therefore expressive language disorder is avoided. However dominant hemispherectomy in adults eliminates expressive language, though they regain automatic verbal responses, diencephalic speech, stock phrases or words and slang words[7,8].

It is now established, on the basis of several studies[4,12,14] that speech centre shifts to right from left in children with left hemisphere lesions or repression of a potential language zone in the right brain occurs.

In the first instance we studied fifteen patients with acquired left-handedness due to right-sided infantile spastic hemiparesis with hypoplasia of the right arm[12]. An initial carotid angiogram excluded vascular anomalies.

Carotid amytal speech test confirmed that the speech centre had shifted to the right hemisphere in 10 out of 15. Every patient was continuously tested for sequence of loss of speech and hemiplegia after Amytal injection and later for recovery of speech or motor power and also for memory of test sentences, objects, names, simple calculations etc. Significantly, there were also two patients who continued to be right-handed despite right hemiparesis but in them the speech centre had shifted to the right side. This finding gave the first clue that a cerebral lesion involving the speech area and not handedness decided shift of centre.

Study and Results

The subjects were 3 male and 2 female patients aged 15 to 25, with flail, wasted or deformed right arm due to polio or injury. They were all previously right-handed and later became left-handed for all habits. There was no family history of left-handedness. The lesion was sustained before the age of eight years in all of them and assessment was done when they were adults. Carotid amytal speech test showed that in all of them the speech centre was still located in the left hemisphere. The details of the Amytal speech test and the battery of neurological and psychological tests done have already been published[12,13].

Discussion

We are not aware of similar language test in such patients by other workers. Scholt in London (1980) has reported on a study of ten patients, with plexus injury and obligatory left handedness. By various tests including linear and circular drawing they found in 7/10 patients, change in direction of lines i.e., left to right, mirror reversal of letters but none had mirror movements. He did not study shift of centre by amytal test. In the book on neurological examination by De Jong

(1979) it is stated that handedness and hemisphere dominance are inherited and that injuries and amputations in childhood may change handedness and possibly also dominance for speech. No details are given.

To quote Subirana (1969) "Shifted dominance: A change in dominance can be brought about by two causes: by a peripheral lesion of the dominant extremity or a central lesion of the dominant hemisphere". Oppenheim's case subsequently discussed by Wernicke relates to an originally right-handed woman who at the age of 17 suffered injury to right hand rendering it useless. Retrained as a left-hander, she later developed a left hemiplegia with receptive aphasia. Lovell (1932) reported another case. A boy with a history of pure right-handedness had his right hand amputated at age 10. After 21 years of left-handedness he developed aphasia resulting from a cyst in the language area of the right hemisphere. These cases illustrate how aphasia can occur with a lesion in the adopted hemisphere, in extracerebral lesions. An Amytal speech test to locate speech centre had not been done in these patients.

In a study from Montreal, among the left-handed, 64 per cent had left cerebral speech centre if it was inherited or primary, whereas in acquired left-handedness, 67 per cent had a right cerebral speech centre[2].

Using visual and auditory evoked potentials in response to flash and click stimuli to predict speech dominance and determining handedness by a questionnaire with 12 criteria, Annett (1967), concluded that handedness was not significantly related to speech dominance especially in those with left-handedness.

Our results suggest that speech centre does not shift if left-handedness is caused by an extracerebral lesion and that it is a cerebral lesion and not handedness that decides the shift.

We have reported earlier the results of neuro-psychological tests in patients with infantile hemiplegia due to cerebral lesions. Twenty patients with right infantile hemiplegia and fifteen with left hemiplegia have been studied by us with various neurological and psychological tests for right and left brain function. With left brain injury in early childhood, non-verbal right brain functions suffer some loss to accommodate the language functions and regain speech. However with right brain injury only non-verbal deficits occur retaining the verbal left brain functions. In either case there is a fall in full scale or total I.Q. Non-verbal functions of the right brain suffered a loss protecting dominant verbal functions with right or left hemiplegia. In the present study of five patients with left-handedness due to extracerebral causes, no such changes were seen because there was no cerebral lesion.

The amytal speech test is 95% accurate in predicting location of the speech centre as judged by speech disturbances after excision of amytal predicted nondominant temporal lobe (Branch 1964). However, more accurate methods by spectral analysis of evoked potentials are also being used[6].

References

1. Annett M (1967) The binominal distribution of right, mixed and left handedness. Q J Exp Psychol 19: 327–333
2. Branch C, Milner B, Rasmusen T (1964) Intracarotid sodium amytal test for the lateralisation of cerebral speech dominance. J Neurosurg 21: 339–405
3. Brain WR (1945) Speech and handedness. Lancet ii: 837–839
4. Baser LS (1962) Hemiplegia of earlier onset and the faculty of speech with special reference to the effects of hemispherectomy. Brain 85: 427–430
5. Dejong RN (1979) The neurological examination, IV Ed. Harper and Row, New York, pp 652
6. Davied AE, Wada JA (1977) Lateralisation of speech dominance: spectral analysis of evoked potentials, J Neurol Neurosurg Psychiatry 40: 1–4
7. Gott PS (1973) Language after dominant hemispherectomy, J Neurol Neurosurg Psychiatry 36: 1082
8. Krynauw RA (1950) Infantile hemiplegia treated by removing one cerebral hemisphere. J Neurol Neurosurg Psychiatry 13: 243
9. Lovell HW, Waggoner RW, Khan EA (1932) Arch Neurol Psychiatry (Chicago) 28: 1179–1182
10. Subirana A (1969) Handedness and cerebral dominance. In: Vinken PJ, Bruyn GW (eds) Handbook of clinical neurology, Vol 4. North Holand, Amsterdam, pp 263–265
11. Srinivasan K (1983) Recovery of intellectual function after injury to young brain. A preliminary report based on a study of patients with infantile hemiplegia. Neurology India 31: 47–49
12. Srinivasan K (1975) A study of infantile hemiplegia with reference to shift of Cerebral speech centre. Neurology India 23: 140–142
13. Schott GD (1980) Mirror movements of left arm following peripheral damage to preferred right arm J Neurol Neurosurg Psychiatry 43: 763–773
14. Teuber H-L (1975) Recovery of functions after brain injury in man-CIBA Symposium 34. Exerpta medica Amsterdam. Elsevier, pp 159–163

Correspondence: Prof. K. Srinivasan, Formerly Head of Neurosciences Department, Madurai Medical College, II.A. By Pass Road, SBI Colony II, Madurai 625016, India.

Acta Neurochirurgica (1993) [Suppl] 56: 85–90

Psychological Mechanisms of Speech Rehabilitation in Aphasic Patients

J. Osman-Sági

Institute of Psychology, Academy of Sciences, Budapest, Hungary

Summary

The theoretical basis of speech rehabilitation and some inherent mechanisms of language/speech, that could be used to overcome speech disorders, are discussed. Among them: Stimulation of speech functions of the right hemisphere, structures of functional systems according to Luria, modular systems in cognitive neuropsychology, and the importance of the use of new processing strategies.

Keywords: Aphasia; rehabilitation.

Introduction

Ever since the phenomenon of aphasia has been known, its treatment is also being attempted. However, the success of speech therapy is a question of contradiction: its pros and cons are still widely discussed in the literature. By many authors the results of speech therapy are considered non-specific, having only a psychotherapeutic effect, while others think improvement of speech in aphasic patients is due to spontaneous recovery. I would like to mention only one of those data that support the hypothesis about the specific learning effect of treatment. The case was published in the Archives of Neurology by Wender in 1989[8].

The author is a professor of classical philology who had lost her knowledge of Latin and Greek after a stroke. She started to relearn Greek with success, but did not study Latin at the time. Two years after the stroke she was able to teach again in Greek, and in the third year, significant difference could be seen between her Greek and Latin knowledge. An experiment was made by her and her colleague, the results of which could be interpreted as an indirect proof of the learning hypothesis. It suggested that in the improvement of her Greek the main role did not belong to spontaneous recovery. In a simple test she was given 10 Greek and 10 Latin words which she could not recall after the stroke. In the following week she was studying the Latin words only, and not the Greek ones. The results of learning were checked a week later. The patient could recognize each of the 10 Latin words, but could not understand the Greek ones. That means therefore, that the Greek words did not come back spontaneously, and the Latin words came back only by learning them.

The problems of the specific treatment techniques and the conditions of their application (in which stages of illness, to which kind of patients etc) are broadly discussed in literature. In this paper I would like to deal a problem which is little treated in the literature of aphasia therapy, that is with the theoretical basis of speech rehabilitation; first of all with some inherent mechanisms of language/speech that could be used to overcome speech disorders after brain damage.

I have selected four aspects of this problem for a short review:

- stimulation of speech functions of the right hemisphere;
- structures of functional systems (Luria);
- modular systems in cognitive neuropsychology;
- processing strategies.

Stimulation of Speech Functions

One of the methods for the treatment of aphasia is stimulation. Stimulation techniques may have three aims:

1. to mobilize the substitutional possibilities of the brain versus speech organization,
2. to stimulate the participation of the right hemisphere in speech functions, and
3. to liberate the functions which are inhibited but not lost. This is called deblocking. (Not only stimulation has a deblocking effect, but other techniques too, like relearning and reorganization. All types of therapy may have a general deblocking effect.)

Stimulation is used mainly for involving speech capabilities of the subdominant hemisphere. The theoretical support to these methods come from the split brain studies by Sperry, Gazzaniga, Zaidel[10] and others who uncovered the specific functions of the subdominant hemisphere in speech[2,9].

The right hemisphere in itself is not able to activate the speech articulation system, since it has no direct access to the motor output. This requires the activation of the Broca area, which is located in the left hemisphere in right-handed people. When the brain is intact the right hemisphere has access to the motor speech output through the corpus callosum. Although in a limited way, the right hemisphere also has its own information processing mechanism for speech comprehension. These processing mechanisms of the two hemispheres are different: the left hemisphere is basically founded on phonematic analysis, that is, the segmentation of the words to sounds, while the right hemisphere is less capable of phonemical-categorical perception of speech sounds, but it has the capacity of global acoustic processing. It can compare the words acoustic patterns to visual ones, thus the more concrete a word, the higher the possibility of the right hemisphere decoding it. That is why the right hemisphere in itself is not able to comprehend syntactical structures, unless they are expressed in lexical units, that is by words and their orders, and not in affixes. Also the right hemisphere will be capable of some reading, provided the text consists of well known words, and comprehension does not need transcoding the letters of each word into phonemes, that is when the words can be recognized only by their global visual configuration. The right hemisphere also takes part in the perception of emotional tones and speech prosody like the intonation. It also plays an important role in the control of sound intensity and pitch levels. The most important speech function of the right hemisphere is that it has an access to the lexicon that is, to the vocabulary. This became very clear when the process of speech comprehension was analysed. At the same time it does not have a short term memory of the same span as the left hemisphere, and it can process the grammatical construction of speech only in a limited way. Thus, the right hemisphere could be used primarily for the stabilization and improvement of the vocabulary. By the stimulation speech prosody it can also be used for the improvement of speech comprehension. A specific feature of the right hemisphere is its understanding written language better than the auditive one, and thus writing and reading can also be utilized for the stimulation or reorganization of speech functions.

There is another way for the right hemisphere to participate in the spontaneous compensation of the damaged speech processes. It is well known that the information processing strategies are different in the two hemispheres. An old problem in neurology is where to "localize" music perception and constructive praxis, or to decide which hemisphere is damaged in acalculia. The split brain studies and the contemporary neuropsychological studies proved that both the left and the right hemispheres participate in these functions. They do this in different ways. The best known approach is that the right hemisphere works in a global way, while the left one processes information in an analytical way. For example in an unknown town we may orientate either by using our visual system only, or by finding orientation points verbally. So the strategies can be very different and can be based on the verbal system to a greater or lesser degree. The activation of the verbal system is one of the main features of the so-called cognitive style. It is evident that cognitive strategies with primary base on the verbal system must be reorganized and restructured after the damage of speech. This may happen in a spontaneous way, but sometimes it may need specific therapy. When the cognitive styles are not fundamentally verbal, the cognitive strategies will usually remain intact and thus can be used for speech therapy more effectively than those based on verbal analysis. Unfortunately the problem of the cognitive style is a little treated field in aphasia therapy.

Using stimulation of speech functions of the right hemisphere there is a fact that we must have in mind, that is the role of the corpus callosum. As Zaidel (1989)[10] and others have shown, the corpus callosum has inhibitory functions first of all; that is, the intensive functioning of the left hemisphere may have an inhibiting effect upon the right one and vice-versa. If we do not pay attention to this fact, we may easily run into deadlock.

Structures of Functional Systems

In the contemporary aphasiology the pioneer of building rehabilitation techniques upon psychological analysis of the speech system was the outstanding Russian neuropsychologist, A.R. Luria. The history of the theoretical development of the aphasia therapy began with his monograph "Traumatic aphasia" published in Russian in 1947. Luria thought that the main method of speech restitution is reorganization and the central idea of his theory was the concept of functional systems.

Luria (1966) characterized the functional systems of each cognitive process from two aspects. The first is that the functional systems are always based on the ontogenetical development of the functions, and he tried to outline a map of the components having part in the cognitive processes. The other aspect is that the functional systems are based upon multimodal sensory inputs. The most quoted example by Luria is the functional system of writing. The articulation of speech has a major role in the development of this system. In the skilled writer the open articulation of speech has no importance in writing, that is in Russian spelling (and so in Hungarian), we use the articulation system only when we have some problems in automatic writing and we have to spell the word. On the other hand, Luria and his co-workers made a study with first-grade school children just learning to write, and their results suggested that the children's spelling would deteriorate if speech articulation was inhibited in any way. This means that even in adults, the structure of the functional system contains certain elements that most probably do not work and do not step automatically into the system, but can be switched on, because originally they formed a part of the functional system.

The other characteristic, as I have already mentioned, is that Luria conceived the functional system as integration of different modalities. In the above mentioned example Luria called attention to the function of the kinaesthetic analyzer, and pointed out that the supplementation of the so-called afferent basis of function is the most important step in the reorganization of the functional systems. According to Luria the first and the most important phase of the rehabilitation process is the analysis of the functional system so as to uncover which particular component is actually damaged in a given cognitive system. For example, if in writing the analysis of the sounds of the words is impaired, then this lost link of the process cannot be substituted by simple copying the visual presentation of the words. If the defect is in the visual analysis, then copying can be one of the best ways of retraining. In neuropsychological rehabilitation as a first step it must be defined which components are intact in a given functional system. The restitution of the functions must be to utilize these components. When we reconstruct a functional system by involving the latent components or by re-organizing the intact elements, then the functional system will be reorganized on an intentional level. This is very important because in the majority of cognitive functions only the beginning of the process is intentional, the rest is automatic. In a later period of therapy the process must be returned back to the automatic

level from this higher level of consciousness and this is one of the major problems in speech therapy.

Modular Systems of Cognitive Neuropsychology

As I mentioned, Luria is considered a forerunner of modern cognitive neuropsychology. Though the Lurian concept of multicomponent functional systems has many features in common with the modular system theory of cognitive neuropsychology, I would like to underline they are not the same. In Luria's functional systems theory a most important idea – I think – is the flexibility of the structure, whereas in the cognitive theory the main idea is that the modules can operate individually and separately; however there are different routes for the same cognitive task. Luria underlined that though the elements of functional systems do work separately as well, they are closely interconnected and interrelated. The theories based on contemporary knowledge of general psychology try to give a schema of the processes of the cognitive functions. The most detailed description of a modular system was done about reading[3,5]. It is well known that in English we have to learn the spelling of the majority of the words, contrary to other languages like Hungarian, Italian, German etc., where we have to learn the general rules of direct phoneme-grapheme transcription. That is, we learn how to decompose words into sounds and phonemes, and learn what letters and graphemes correspond to them. Exceptions are infrequent. In English there are two ways of reading. One of them is relying on the meaning of the word. The written word – without segmentation – has a direct access to the meaning. The other way is analysing words letter by letter, and this way finding their meaning. These two ways of reading can be injured separately. The direct access to the meaning of the words can be impaired, that is the patient recognizes the written word globally without being able to analyse it letter by letter, and still understands its meaning. This is called deep dyslexia in English literature. The other groups of patients can only read by analysing words letter by letter. Deep dyslexic Hungarian patients are unable to read suffixes and affixes connected to the words. When recognizing the word stems only, they will make grammatical errors.

Figure 1 illustrates a part of the best known map of a modular system in neuropsychology. The impaired routes in both types of dyslexia can be discovered in this map: in cases of deep dyslexia the defect must be somewhere between the visual input lexicon and the semantic system. In the other type of reading distur-

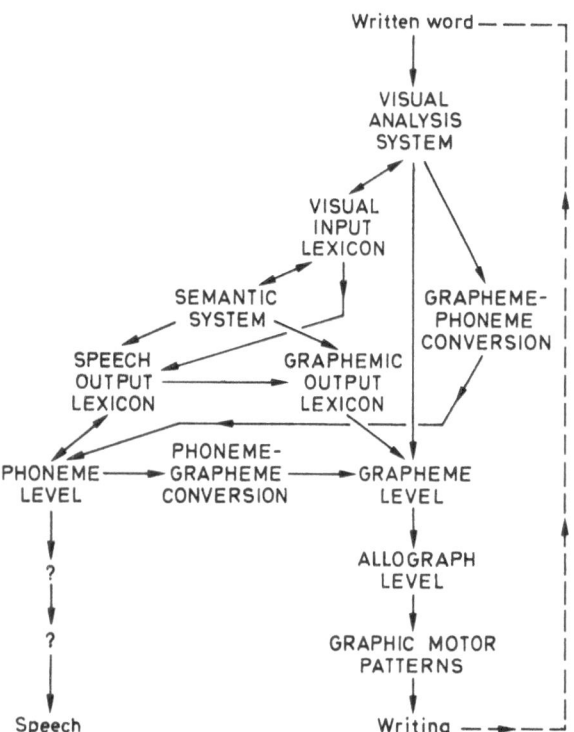

Fig. 1. Part of the "map" of reading from the model of single word recognition by Ellis A, Young A (1988) in "Human Cognitive Neuropsychology"

bance – when the patients can read only with grapheme/phoneme conversion – it may happen that the system of the visual analysis is what is impaired.

Processing Strategies

It is obvious that reading may function normally if based on the intact paths and modules. However, this does not mean that the activated route is the only one to be followed, but it means that based on it other means have to be retaught. When we talk about the methodological problems of rehabilitation or about the inner psychological mechanisms of recovery we always emphasize that during recovery the brain does not create new structures, but uses new strategies. How can this be interpreted? One of the meanings of the strategy was already mentioned when talking about cognitive style in connection with the right hemisphere. In information-processing other strategies are also possible. Among these I would like to enter into details of the sentence comprehension strategies.

The experimental study of this problem was done in a cross-linguistic research project in eight languages. It was organized by Bates E. (Univ. of California, San Diego) and McWhinney B. (Carnegie–Mellon Univ., Pittsburgh).

For understanding a sentence we have to know who the agent is, what the agent aims at, that is, which of the nouns is the subject and which of the nouns is the object of a given sentence. The sentence itself contains different references, different cues to do that. In English language one of the case references is the word order. The place of direct object is always after the verb, and the agent usually stands in front of it. In German and Italian the importance of the word order is much smaller but in these languages the semantic features of the agent (being animated or neutral) plays a more important role. Thus in English the word order will clearly show which nouns will be the subject and object of a sentence, while in other languages we have to lean on other cues when decoding a sentence. In Hungarian in a simple sentence like "the boy is chasing the dog" the affix of the direct object is the only information to make this distinction. The word order and the subject's animacy have no importance in healthy people.

The so called "enactment task" used in this study was set up in the following way: two little toys were put in front of the patient like e.g. a dog and a chair. The patient was instructed to enact with these toys the sentence spoken by the examiner, e.g. "the dog jumps over the chair" or "the chair jumps over the dog". Some of the sentences were not correct grammatically, because the affixes of the direct object were missing. The word order was also varied. In Hungarian language word order is free, but we usually use a so called canonical word order (subject-verb-object), or sometimes subject-object-verb. In the Hungarian language there are no morphological signs to show whether or not the subject is animated. We have made 54 sentences. Each sentence consisted of two nouns and one verb. Variables were the following: patient's groups (Broca's-, Wernicke's-, and anomic aphasics and healthy people), word order, the animacy of the nouns, and the place of the noun with a direct object marker affix. We analysed which noun was selected by the patient as the agent, the first one or the second one pronounced. The results are given in percentage of how many times the patient chooses the first noun as agent in his response.

Figure 2 shows the results of English, German and Italian experiments after Bates, Friederici, and Wulfeck (1987)[1] as well as the Hungarian ones. In English it is quite clear that word order determines completely which noun is selected as agent in the healthy group. Word order has a similar effect in a smaller degree in English aphasic patients. This effect is much smaller

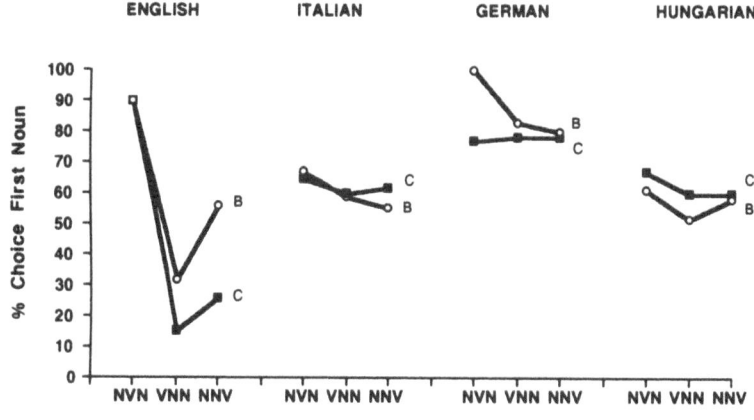

Fig. 2. Effect of word order on selection of the first noun as agent in Broca's aphasic patients (*B*) and control group (*C*) (*N* = noun, *V* = verb)

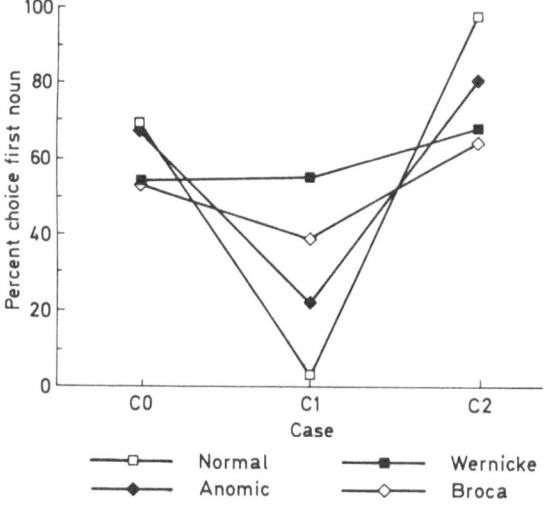

Fig. 3. Effect of the place of case marker on the first noun selection in Hungarian. *C1* = direct object case marker on the first noun, that means the second noun is the agent of the sentence. *C2* = direct object marker on the second noun, the agent is the first noun. *C0* = no case marker in the sentence. That means the sentence is ungrammatical

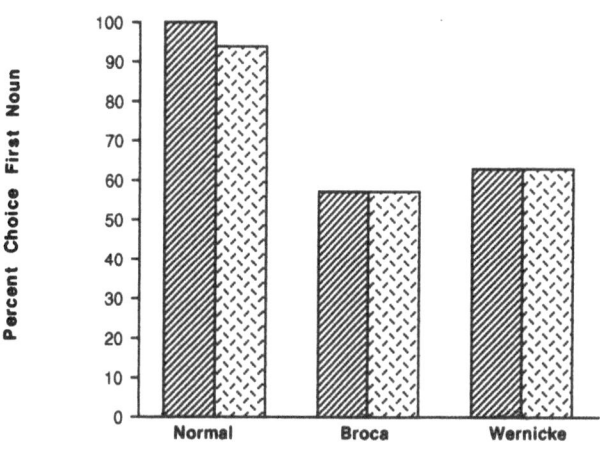

Fig. 4. Results of Hungarian aphasic patients and control group in two conditions of variables interactions

both in German and Italian, and in Hungarian as well. If we analyse the interaction of word order and case marking, we can see that word order has little influence on which noun was selected as agent, but contrary to this fact the case-suffix does. If we analyse the effect of the agent being animate or inanimate, we come to similar results: animacy in itself has no influence on the person's strategy, it is the affix of the object that will determine which noun is the subject and which one is the object. When the affix of the object is not present then both word order and animacy will have a more pronounced effect. It has to be mentioned that contrary to the generally accepted view, the Hungarian results (MacWhinney, Osman-Sagi, and Slobin, 1991) suggest that the Broca's aphasic patients are not the only ones

who have difficulties with grammar, the Wernicke's aphasic patients are less able than the Broca's to use the affixes for processing direct objects in sentence comprehension (Fig. 3).

Comparing the patients' strategies (Fig. 4) the following could be observed: if in the sentence there is a direct object affix on the second noun (*C2*), that is, the basic cue is present, but the other two conditions provide minimal information – the word order is not canonical (*VNN* condition) and both nouns are animated (*AA*), the percentage of first noun choices are the same in Broca's group of patients and the Wernicke's group of patients as in the sentences when the direct object affix is not present (*C0*), but the word order is canonical (*NVN*), and the first noun is animated (*AI*). Effect of convergency of these two optimal conditions – which are not crucial cues in Hungarian – do not differ from strategy which uses the direct object affix alone.

Thus the different strategies may well be used during the process of therapy, that is when the patient is unable to use the direct object affix as the main cue for decoding, but is able to use word order and the semantic feature of animacy as thus, then with the help of these means the direct object affix, whose processing was impaired, may have recovered and be utilized.

References

1. Bates E, Friederici A, Wulfeck B (1987) Comprehension in aphasia: A cross-linguistic study. Brain and Language 32: 19–67
2. Code C (1987) Language, aphasia and the right hemisphere. John Wiley, Chichester
3. Coltheart M, Patterson KE, Marshall JC (eds) (1980) Deep dyslexia. Routledge & Kegan, London
4. Coltheart M, Sartori G, Job R (1987) The cognitive neuropsychology of language. Lawrence Erlbaum, Hillsdale
5. Ellis AW (ed) (1982) Normality and pathology in cognitive functions. Academic Press, London
6. Luria AR (1947) Traumatic aphasia. Izd Akad Med Nauk SSSR, Moskow (Russian)
7. Luria AR (1962) Higher cortical functions in man. Moscow Univ. Press, Moscow (Russian)
8. Wender D (1989) Aphasic victim as investigator. Arch Neurol 46: 91–92
9. Young AW (ed) (1983) Functions of the right hemisphere. Academic Press, London
10. Zaidel E (1989) Hemispheric independence as a paradigm case for cognitive neuroscience. Paper presented at 12th European Conference of International Neuropsychological Society. Antwerp

Correspondence: J. Osman-Sági, Institute of Psychology, Academy of Sciences, Budapest, Hungary.

Acta Neurochirurgica (1993) [Suppl] 56: 91–95

Features of Computer Language: Communication of Computers and Its Complexity

L. Lovász

Department of Computer Science, Eötvös Lóránd University, Budapest, Hungary; and Princeton University, New Jersey, USA

Summary

Motivated by computer science, in particular, by applications to data security, electronic correspondance and cryptography, interactive proofs extend the 2000 years old, well established notion of mathematical proof. The key to these development is *complexity* which is defined as the minimum amount of a certain resource needed to complete a computational task. In this paper, the idea of an interactive proof system and its application in computer science is illuminated on everyday examples, without giving technical details.

Keywords: Complexity, interactive proof, zero-knowledge proof, passward scheme.

Introduction

Recent developments in the theory of computing constitute a novel branch of mathematics and no doubt these mathematical ideas and tools may prove as important in the life sciences as the tools of classical mathematics (calculus and algebra) have proved in physics and chemistry. The key notion in the theory of computing is that of the *complexity*. The brain, being probably the most complex organ both structurally and functionally, seems to be particularly suited for investigation from this point of view.

Computer science, also called *informatics*, is often defined as the theory of storing, processing, and communicating information. These aspects (and their variations) lead to various measures of complexity. We may speak of the complexity of a structure, meaning the amount of information (number of bits) in the most economical "blueprint" of the structure; this is the minimum space we need to store enough information about the structure that allows us its reconstruction. We may also speak of the algorithmic complexity of a certain task: this is the minimum time needed to carry out this task on a computer. And we may also speak

of the communication complexity of tasks involving more than one processor: this is the number of bits that have to be transmitted in solving this task.

It is important that this notion can be defined and measured in a mathematically precise way. The resulting theory is as exact as Euclidean geometry and, at the same time, plays its role in the study of a large variety of phenomena, from computers to genetics to statistical mechanics (and, I hope, in brain research!). The elaboration of the mathematical theory would, of course, be beyond the scope of this talk. Garey and Johnson (1979) give an introduction to some aspects of the theory; Babai (1990)[2] gives a mathematical but very enjoyable introduction and survey, along with a discussion of some of the ethical issues raised by the more and more wide-spread use of electronic pre-publication. I will try here to illuminate by everyday examples some of the recent developments in the field, and will show the "logic" of what is happening.

How to Save the Last Move in Chess?

Alice and Bob are playing chess over the phone. They want to interrupt the game for the night; how can they do it so that the person to move should not get the improper advantage of being able to think about his move whole night? At a tournament, the last move is not made on the board, only written down, put in an envelope, and deposited with the referee. But now the two players have no referee, no envelope, no contact other than the telephone line. The player making the last move (say, Alice) has to tell something; but this information should not be enough to determine the move, or else Bob would gain undue advantage. The next morning (or whenever they continue the game) she has to give some additional information, some "key", which allows Bob to reconstruct the move.

But this seems to be impossible. If she gives enough information the first time to uniquely determine her move, Bob will know the move; if the information given the first time allows several moves, then she can think about it overnight, figure out the best among these, and give this remaining information, the "key", accordingly.

If we measure information in the sense of classical information theory, then there is no way out of this dilemma. But complexity comes to our help: it is not enough to communicate information, it must also be processed.

To describe a solution, we need a little preparation from mathematics. *Prime numbers* are those positive integers larger than 1 that cannot be written as the product of two smaller positive integers: 2, 3, 5, 7, 11, 13, ... There are infinitely many such numbers; there are prime numbers with any given number of digits; in fact, we can find prime numbers with a prescribed number of digits and up to a third of the digits also prescribed. Here I mean "we can find" also in the sense that rather efficient computer programs exist to test if a given integer is a prime, and also to generate primes. These programs can be used to extend, say, a 4-digit number to a prime number with 200 digits, using a moderate-size computer.

Euclid already knew that every positive integer can be written as the product of prime numbers (e.g. $30 = 2 \times 3 \times 5$), and this decomposition is unique. But until now, no efficient way is known to *find* such a decomposition. Of course, very powerful supercomputers and massively parallel systems can be used to find decompositions by brute force for fairly large numbers; the current limit is around a 100 digits, and the difficulty grows very fast (exponentially) with number of digits. To find the prime decomposition of a number with 400 digits is way beyond the possibilities of computers in the foreseeable future.

Returning to our problem, Alice and Bob can agree to encode every move as a 4-digit number (say, "11" means "K", "6" means "f", and "3" means itself, so "1163" means "Kf3"). Alice extends these four digits to a prime number "1163..." with 200 digits. She also generates another prime with 201 digits, computes the product of them (this would take rather long on paper, but is trivial using even a personal computer). The result is a number N with 400 or 401 digits; she sends this number to Bob. Next morning, she sends both prime factors to Bob. He checks that they are primes

and that their product is N, and reconstructs Alice's move from the first four digits of the smaller prime.

The number N contains all the information about her move: this consists of the first for digits of the smaller prime factor of N. Alice has to commit herself to the move when sending N. The rest of the smaller prime factor and the other prime factor serve as an "envelope": they hide the actual information from Bob. To find out Alice's move Bob would have to find the prime factors of N; this is, however, hopeless. So Bob only learns the move when the factors are revealed the next morning.

What Alice and Bob have established is an electronic "notary public": a method to deposit information at a certain time that can be retrieved at a given later time. The key ingredient of their scheme is *complexity*: the computational difficulty to find the factors of an integer. Such a scheme, and similar schemes like electronic authorization, authentication, signatures, passwords, etc. are extremely important in computer security, cryptography, and a number of other fields. It is even more surprising that these developments inspired fundamental changes in notions at the very heart of mathematics, such as in the 2000 year old notion of a *proof*. Let us sketch the road that leads to these changes.

How to Check a Password – Without Knowing It?

In a bank, a cash machine works by name and password. This system is safe as long as the password is kept secret. But there is one weak point in security: the computer of the bank must store the password, and the programmer may learn it and later misuse it.

Complexity theory provides a scheme where the bank can verify that the customer does indeed know the password – without storing the password itself. One solution uses the same construction as our telephone chess example. The password is a 200-digit prime number P (this is, of course, too long for everyday use, but it illustrates the idea best). When the customer chooses the password, he also chooses another prime with 201 digits, forms the product N of the two primes, and tells the bank the number N. When the teller is used, the customer tells his name and the password P. The computer of the bank checks whether or not P is a divisor of N; if so, it accepts P as a proper password. The division of a 400 digit number by a 200 digit number is a trivial task for a computer.

Let us assume now that a programmer learns the number N stored along with the files of our customer. To use this in order to impersonate the customer, he

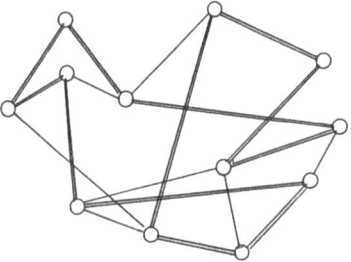

Fig. 1. A graph and a Hamilton cycle

has to find a 200-digit number that is a divisor of N; but this is essentially the same problem as finding the prime factorization of N, and, as remarked above, is hopelessly difficult. So – even though all the necessary information is contained in the number N – the computational complexity of the factoring problem protects the password of the custumer!

There are many other schemes to achieve the same. Let us describe another one that we shall also need later. A *graph* is a figure composed of *nodes* (denoted by points in the plane) and *edges* (denoted by segments connecting certain pairs of nodes). A *Hamilton cycle* in the graph is a closed polygon that goes through every node exactly once. Figure 1 shows a graph in which a Hamilton cycle is marked.

We can use this notion for a password scheme as follows. The customer chooses a polygon H on 200 nodes (labelled $1, 2, \ldots, 200$) as his password (this means that the password is a certain ordering of these labels, like $(7, 50, 1, \ldots, 197, 20, 3)$). Then he adds some further edges randomly, and gives the resulting graph G to the bank (it is a difficult question how many further edges to add, and from what distribution, to hide the Hamilton cycle best; but we ignore this issue here). When the customer uses the teller, the computer simply checks that every edge of the polygon encoded by the password is an edge of the graph G stored for the given customer, and if this checks out, it accepts the passwords.

The safety of this scheme depends on the fact that given a graph G with a few hundred nodes (and with an appropriate number of edges), it is hopelessly difficult to find a Hamilton cycle in it (even if we know that it exists). Many other problems in mathematics could be used in password schemes: e.g., the bank may store a system of equations, and the password could be a solution; or the bank may store a graph, and the password may be a given number of nodes, mutually connected by edges etc. The security depends on the difficulty (computational complexity) of *finding* this solution. There is a theory, central to theoretical com-

puter science, that provides means to measure this difficulty and thereby distinguish "difficult" and "easy" problems. The Hamilton cycle problem, or the problem of finding a solution to a system of quadratic equations, are among the most difficult (so yield in a sense the safest schemes); the problem of solving linear equations is easy (and so it would give an insecure scheme), while the problem of factoring an integer is "in between". The exact definitions needed for the exact statement of the results are beyond the scope of this paper; we refer to Garey and Johnson (1979) for a technical treatment.

How to Use Your Password – Without Telling It?

The password scheme discussed in the previous section is secure if the program is surely correct; but what happens if the program itself contains a part that simply reads off the password the costumer uses, and tells it to the programmer? In this case, the password is compromised if it is used but once. There does not seem to be any way out – how could one use the passport without giving it to the computer?

It sounds paradoxical, but *there is a scheme which allows the customer to convince the bank that he knows the password – without giving the slightest hint as to what the password is*! I'll give an informal description of the idea (following Blum 1987), by changing roles: let me be the customer and you (the audience) play the role of the computer of the bank. I'll use two overhead projectors. The graph G shown on the first projector is the graph known to the bank; I label its nodes for convenience. My password is a Hamilton cycle (a polygon going through each node exactly once) in this graph, which I know but don't want to reveal.

I have prepared two further transparencies. The first contains a polygon with the same number of nodes as G, drawn with random positions for the nodes and without labels. The second transparency, overlayed the first, contains the labels of the nodes and the edges that complete it to a drawing of the graph G (with the nodes in different positions). The two transparencies are covered by a sheet of paper.

Now the audience may choose: should I remove the top sheet or the two top sheets? No matter which choice is made, the view contains no information about the Hamilton cycle, since it can be predicted: if the top sheet is removed, what is shown is a re-drawing of the graph G, with its nodes in random positions; if the two top sheets are removed, what is shown is a polygon with the right number of nodes, randomly drawn in the plane (Fig. 2), but since this view does not include the

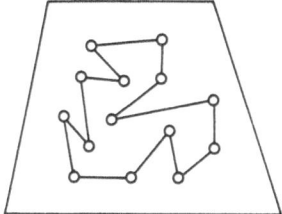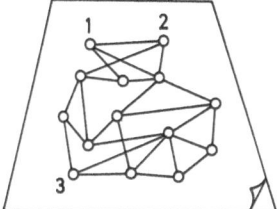

Fig. 2. Zero-knowledge proof of the existence of a Hamilton cycle

labels of the nodes, it does not tell how this polygon lies in the original picture. And the two views are *not* shown together!

But the audience does gain information from the fact that *it sees what is expected*. This is an evidence for my knowing a Hamilton cycle in *G*! For suppose that *G* contains no Hamilton cycle, or if it does, I don't know this cycle. How can I prepare the two transparencies? Either I cheat by drawing something different on the bottom transparency (a polygon with fewer nodes, or missing edges), or by having a different graph on the two transparencies together.

Of course, I may be lucky (say, I draw a polygon with fewer edges and the audience opts to view the two transparencies together) and I will not be discovered; but if I cheat, I only have a chance of 1/2 to get away with it. We can repeat this 100 times (each time with a brand new drawing!); then my chance for being lucky each time is less than 2^{-100}, which is much less than the probability that a meteorite hits the building during this demonstration. So if a 100 times in a row, the audience sees what it expects, this is a *proof* that I know a Hamilton cycle in the graph!

The most interesting aspect of the scheme described above is that it extends the notion of a *proof*, thought (at least in mathematics) to be well established for more than 2000 years. In the classical sense, a proof is written down entirely, and then it is verified by the reader. Here, there is *interaction* between the prover and the verifier: the action taken by the prover depends on "questions" by the verifier. The notion of interactive proof systems was introduced independently by Goldwasser et al. (1985)[9] and by Babai (1985)[1], and has led to many deep and surprising results in computer science and mathematical logic. The above scheme is only one kind of the uses of interaction; it is called a *zero knowledge proof* (not to be comfused with some university exams!), and was *introduced by Goldwasser et al. (1985)*, and extended by Goldreich et al. (1986)[8].

How to Handle Submissions that Keep the Main Results Secret?

Our next two examples come from a field which causes much headache to many of us: editing scientific journals. These are "fun" examples and their purpose is to illuminate the logic of interactive proofs rather than propose real-life applications (although with the fast development of e-mail, electronic bulletin boards, on-line reviewing, and other forms of electronic publications – who knows?).

A typical impasse situation in journal editing is caused by the following letter: "I have a proof of Fermat's Last Theorem, but I won't send you the details because I am afraid you'll steal it. But I want you to announce the result". All we can do is to point out that the policy of the Journal is to publish results only together with their proofs (whose correctness is verified by two referees). There is no way to guarantee that the editor and/or the referee, having read the proof, does not publish it under his own name (unfortunately, this does seem to happen occasionally).

The result sketched in the previous chapter, however, can resolve the dilemma. One feels that the situation is similar: the author has to convince the editor that he has a proof, without giving any information about the details of the proof. Now there is a general result by Cook, Karp and Levin, which, in our case, gives the following: for every mathematical statement *T* and number *k* one can construct a graph *G* such that *T* has a proof of length at most *k* if and only if *G* has a Hamilton cycle. Moreover, the size of the graph is not too large (bounded by k^2). So the editor can come up with the following suggestion upon receiving the above letter: "Please construct the graph corresponding to Fermat's last theorem and the length of your proof, and prove me, using Blum's protocol, that this graph has a Hamilton cycle". This takes some interaction (exchange of correspondence), but in principle it can be done.

How to Referee Exponentially Long Papers?

But of course, the real difficulty with editing a Journal is to find referees, especially for longer papers. Who wants to spend months to read a paper of, say, 150 pages, and look for errors in the complicated formulas filling its pages? And, unfortunately, the devil is often hidden in the little details: a "−" instead of a "+" on the 79-th page may spoil the whole paper....

Recent results in the theory of interactive proofs offer new possibilities. A flow of results[4,12,13] has shown that the power of interaction is far larger than previously believed; it may reduce the length of a "proof" (roughly speaking) to its logarithm!

As an example, assume that a chess player with supernatural powers discovers that white always wins if he plays properly. How does she convince the world about this? To analyze a chess game from the beginning, going through all possible sequences of moves would take more time than the duration of the universe. But these recent results about interactive proofs would make it possible for her to convince everybody that she always wins with white – in a few thousand steps. (One possible interactive proof scheme is simply play a game and see who wins. But since almost everybody beats me no matter who is white, this interactive proof is not very convincing.)

The results are too technical to even state them without proof (and the proof is difficult), but I try to give an idea of one of them (see Babai (1990)[2] for a more detailed but still very enjoyable presentation). It is commonplace in mathematics that sometimes making a proof longer (including more detail and explanation) makes it easier to read. Can this be measured? If a proof is written down compactly, without redundancy, then one has to read the whole proof in order to check its correctness. One way of interpreting the results mentioned above is that there is a way to write down a proof so that a referee can check its correctness by reading only a tiny fraction of it. The proof becomes longer than necessary, but not much longer. The number of characters the referee has to read is only about the *logarithm* of the original proof length! To be precise, if the original proof has length N then the new proof can be checked by reading $\log N \log \log N$ characters; see Feige et al. (1991)[7]. So a 2000-page proof (and such proofs exist!), having about 2^{25} bits, can be checked by reading about $25.5 = 125$ characters, or less than 2 lines!

This modified write-up of the proof may be viewed as an "encoding"; the encoding protects against "local" errors just like classical error-correcting codes protect against "local" errors in telecommunication. The novelty here is the combination of ideas from error-correcting codes with complexity theory.

Complexity theory enters most of the fundamental questions of information theory: the difficulty of coding/decoding, generating and recognizing randomness, the power of interaction in various tasks etc. It is natural to expect that complexity theory will also play an important role in the life sciences, in understanding, among others, the genetic code, the living being as a unit, or the brain.

References

1. Babai L (1985) Trading group theory for randomness. In: Proc 17th ACM Symp Theory of Computing, pp 421–429
2. Babai L (1990) E-mail and the unexpected power of interaction. In: Proc 5th Ann Structure in Complexity Theory Conference. IEEE, New York, pp 30–44
3. Babai L, Fortnow L, Levin L, Szegedy M (1991) Checking computations in polylogarithmic time. In: Proc 23rd ACM Symp Theory of Computing, pp 21–31
4. Babai L, Fortnow L, Lund C (1990) Non-deterministic exponential time has two-prover interactive protocols. In: Proc 31st Ann Symp Foundations of Computer Science, IEEE, New York, pp 16–25
5. Blum M (1987) How to prove a theorem so no one else can claim it. In: Gleason AM (ed) Proc Int Congress of Math 1986. Am Math Soc, pp 1444–1451
6. Cook SA (1971) The complexity of theorem proving procedures. Proc 3rd Ann ACM Symp Theory of Computing (Shaker Heights, 1971). ACM, New York, pp 151–158
7. Feige U, Goldwasser S, Lovász L, Safra S, Szegedy M (1991) Approximating clique is almost NP-complete. In: 32nd Ann Symp Foundations of Computer Science. IEEE, New York
8. Goldreich O, Micali S, Wigderson A (1986) Proofs that yield nothing but the validity of the assertion, and a methodology of cryptographic protocol design. Proc 27th Ann Symp Foundations of Computer Science. IEEE, New York, pp 174–187
9. Goldwasser S, Micali S, Rackoff C (1985) The knowledge complexity of interactive proof systems. In: Proc 17th ACM Symp Theory of Computing, ACM, New York, pp 291–304
10. Karp RM (1972) Reducibility among combinatorial problems. In: Miller RE, Thatcher JW (eds) Complexity of Computer Computations, Plenum Press, pp 85–103
11. Levin L (1972) Universal'nyĭe perebornyĭe zadachi (Universal search problems: in Russian), Problemy Peredachi Informatsii 9: 265–266
12. Lund C, Fortnow L, Karloff H, Nisan N (1990) Algebraic methods for interactive proof systems. In: Proc 31st Ann Symp Foundations of Computer Science. IEEE, New York, pp 2–10
13. Shamir A, IP = PSPACE. Proc 31st Ann Symp Foundations of Computer Science. IEEE, New York, pp 11–15
14. Yao A (1986) How to generate and exchange secrets. Proc 27th Ann Symp Foundations of Computer Science. IEEE, New York, pp 162–167

Correspondence: L. Lovász, Department of Computer Science, Princeton University, Princeton, NJ 08544, U.S.A.

Acta Neurochirurgica (1993) [Suppl] 56: 96–99

Computer and the Thought Process

T. Vámos

Computer and Automation Institute, Academy of Sciences, Budapest, Hungary

Summary

Modelling of brain is an eternal problem and was revitalized by arrogant claims of some computer scientists. Several basic results of mathematics, especially in problems of uncertainty, computational complexity and logic prove limits of computation and indications that the brain works otherwise. The complexity of brain is not accessible by current electronic technology. However, brain research and computer science can learn a lot from each other by revealing relevant analogies.

Keywords: Brain research, modelling, computer science, artificial intelligence, cognitive psychology.

Introduction

I approach our common problems from three points of view:

1) modelling the brain by computers,
2) using analogies of the brain in computer science,
3) cognitive processes and computer methods.

All three started very early, much before the computers or modern medical science. The problem whether a brain could be substituted by a mechanism had a flourishing period in the Age of Reason, d'Alembert, Descartes, several other philosophers and natural scientists raised pros and cons; the celebrated Turing test was virtually invented by Descartes. He used the idea for discriminating between the human and the animal mind and the opinion advocated that only the latter can have a machine surrogate – but it can!

Creating conceptual machines is an old story as well, by using logic or other means of human reasoning for the "computation" of consequences, conceptual relations. The Chinese oracle of I Ching or the rotational disks of Raymond Lullus (13–14th c.) are representatives of the idea, but we find a deep hint at Artificial Intelligence-like thinking in the notes of Lady Ada, Byron's daughter who worked for Babbage and is considered to have been the first computer programmer.

A very modern idea about the cognitive processes, or not too different from the same – as observable from the attitude of our cognitive psychology – can be found in the works of Ibn Sina (Avicenna).

These are only snapshots of the past of these ideas. Similarly to each notion in human intellectual development, they have a long history, celebrated and forgotten antecedents; constructed and created consciously and unconsciously, having followed or denied their masters.

This introduction should not serve as a pedantic exhibition but only as a warning for the continuity and volatility of firm knowledge. Although we know a lot more than our ancestors, we cannot say that we are so much nearer to any final truth (if such exists at all).

Brain-Machine Model

Especially after the rapid development of electronic circuits and computers we see a proliferation of neural and brain models, theories about the brain's activity structures based on computer metaphors. The Perceptron, the McCullogh-Pitts model were modest attempts but the last hullabaloo, the neural nets and computation appear much more arrogant in some people's claims. The original ambition of Artificial Intelligence was the same, a perfect model and based on that the incoming ability of a perfect substitution which should be much better than the natural mind. We can quote Simon and Newell about their General Problem Solver and predictions for the near future which expired long ago.

The other side was marked by John von Neumann himself and by philosophers like H. Putnam, H.L. Dreyfus and S. Dreyfus.

The key issue here is complexity and the simplified answer is that the brain does it otherwise – the latter being the subject of Sects. 2 and 3. The comparison data of the human brain and the most powerful computers are well-known, we should not quote them before this professional community. There are several other reasons for this kind of inadequacy on the computer side. This can be classified in two groups. The classification is artificial and somehow arbitrary as any other, but it is based just on the problems of the methods used by computer science. The first is the complexity in a strong sense and its consequence, the combinatorial explosion. Any system and therefore any task modelled by the system – if it has more than trivial components – exhibits behavior much beyond any physically realizable capacities of computers. Any ordering problem of a high number of actors, pieces, with a similarly higher number of constraints is of this class, e.g. the famous travelling salesman problem where an optimal travelling schedule should be designed for a great number of widely dispersed cities. Similar complex problems are the search for an optimal chess strategy, the breaking of sophisticated codes etc., many problems which look like artificial, complicated exercises but are really simplified models of real life tasks. These are linear systems; we did not calculate the effects of nonlinearities, chaotic behavior and several other factors which are not modelled by a linear system. Uncertainty, stochastic behavior, the changes of these uncertainties during time multiply this incomputable complexity by many orders of magnitude.

The second is deeply lying in the methods used for computation but the background is even deeper. We apply a few computational-mathematical disciplines in our models for computer processing. One group is devoted to the uncertainty itself. The original probability methods have now a great number of competing procedures for the same, never completely solvable and never completely satisfiable problem of uncertainty calculations. The transitory firm belief in statistics-based probability calculus is over, we know how much all these statistics are dependent of the initial hypotheses, prejudices, how limited is the *a posteriori* knowledge based on statistics and probability calculus for *a priori* decisions. As mentioned before, uncertainty multiplies the complexity by orders of magnitude.

The uncertainty of data and the uncertainty of relation of these uncertain data is treated by logic. This is a basic contradiction of any human but more of any computer reasoning: logic operates in a closed (rational, logical) world where no contradiction exists, each datum, fact, consequence is reachable from the others by graphs of logic, i.e. by the Law of Reason. In this world a few basic facts and relations are the final bricks and mortars of the edifice of the Universe. You encountered several similar hypotheses in biology: the primitive models of the neurons and the initial picture of the genetic code.

This world is reduced to ruins. The non-existence of a closed world is proved first in mathematics and then in any conceptual structure. Logic is a practical device, if it is used in an appropriate, limited way but not as a general problem-solver. The openness of the general or of any complex problem opens the computer problem-solver towards the incomputable space of high complexity. What we do now is an extremely modest attempt: delimit a very narrow field of problems (e.g. one special medical diagnostic task) and use it as a support for human action, not with the goal of substituting the human operator. Where we can do it (e.g. some process controls, banking operations etc.) we feel the limits at any slightly exceptional case. This is not so bad, we can use our cars but we never think about substituting our legs – the metaphor is characteristic but the brain-computer relation is much further!

All arrogant claims of Artificial Intelligence – human quality machine translation, recognition of continuous spoken text or ordinary handwriting, reaching the level of the world master in chess, machine expertise in any profession better than human – have failed until now and should fail in the future because of a different ability of fighting complexity and therefore a different ability of problem solving. The two developments, the brain and the machine, had and have a different course – they are in several aspects diverging and not converging; this means that computers can be used in brain modelling only in a very limited – but sometimes practical – way, and just because of the major differences the brain and the machine can create an excellent coexistence.

Machine as a Brain Model

The opposite substitution is weak as well. We can draw some weak analogies, it helps in a way of understanding the required technological processes as memory, memory organization, recognition, sensory input, etc. but going further or taking the analogies as solution methods is misleading.

We can iterate several arguments of the other issue – of the brain-computer relation. As brain research is progressing, it finds more and more specific, variable functions, changing, adapting behavior, nonsynaptic connections, a fantastic complexity of electrical, chemical, developmental, organic functions which have no simile in our computer technology, any model of those is an oversimplification. I can admire the naïve belief – or disdain the arrogant advertisements – which is expressed by these claims. However, there are several lessons of the brain's structure and activity which can be useful in computer science if used in a humble and critical way. The first analogy is the trivial functional classification: input-output, memory, processing, access to different levels of memory as mentioned before. However, the continuation of this analogic way of function matching is misleading because of the enumerated reasons. The main focus of interest is really the secret, how the human brain solves problems which are unsolvable for the devices of technology and whether we can learn anything discovering even parts of this puzzle.

A continuous trend in technology is to approximate the complexity of the brain, i.e. increase the number of active components and their possible interconnections. In spite of the dramatic progress in this field we see now the physical limitations of the semiconductor devices used until now, and we can say that this way cannot lead to the same functional compactness as the living cells achieved at their molecular level. A molecular computer, if it can be created, is something completely different from our present organizations, it has to consider some stochastic behavior instead of the highly reliable components of the computers used now – a different philosophy as nature is different from our artifacts. The major problem what we are looking at is the highly distributed and highly parallel features of the brain. This is a lesson which is relevant for us and our recent systems are developing in these directions although the ways how technical systems do it are different: less flexible, less adaptive, less versatile in one way, i.e. in the "hardware" operation but more the same in another, the natural brain being a result of development of hundreds of millions of years; a computer on the other hand is a utensil designed for practical present-day use and obsolete after 3–4 years. I think it would be crazy, if anybody would interchange the two developments. We do not interchange our eyes or those of the beloved partner with the best omniscient cameras.

Here I mention two further issues. The first relates to a brain-imitating nomenclature of a technological trend: neural computer. These are really parallel processing, rather distributed devices based on a very simplistic neuron analogue (much more simplistic than the original Bohr model of atoms compared to the

real atomic structure) and some simple, long-known connection and algorithmic ideas. They are practical devices, especially after some technological maturation, mostly as parts of conventional computing systems, they can be used especially for pattern recognition but are very far from any imitation of the brain, any breakthrough in intelligence. No task is demonstrated – even not by a theoretical thought experiment – which could be solved by them and not by any present serial-mode commercial computer. They can offer only some practical partial solutions.

The other issue is very important. Having understood the basic differences between man and machine we started to think about an ideal man-machine symbiosis where man has the unquestionable priority and the machine should be adjusted to the requirements convenience, attitudes and goals of humans. This means ergonomy, user-friendly software, human-oriented, computer-supported operation and cooperation, task definition and organization. I firmly believe – and this conviction is shared by many other colleagues of my field – that computers should and shall contribute to a more human-oriented and humanistic life, just the opposite of several sci-fi nightmares or present culturally disqualifying trends.

Cognitive Lessons

The last topic is a lesson after the two preceding ones. Having acknowledged the limitations of our mathematico-logical tools and of our hardware capacities we returned to be humble learners of human and animal cognitive processes and investigators of the optimal cooperation between man and machine. I emphasize the animal's neural system and cognition as well, we learnt how wonderful this works in those tasks which were relevant in their development and adaptation, sometimes much better than the human one, not speaking about the computers. No robot or no acrobat can attain the movement-control abilities of a cat or no analytical device can match the scent-based chemical pattern recognition of a dog. These are not only due to very special input-output devices but have their background in the brain. All recent results of cognitive psychology indicate that the brain is not a computer, it is not a statistico-logical machine, it works many times against all these exact rules – and it works.

We find behind these phenomena patterns, Gestalts, schemes, somehow related entities, stored, compressed and connected in a mystical way and patterns of the dynamics of these patterns, how they extend their scope, how they do connections, how they change their special, local metric. Emotions are discovered to be one of the stimuli of these dynamic changes in patterns and pattern relations. Research is focused on these lessons; my own group's interest is specially oriented to the problems, how we can use what we learn about decision making of human experts of different fields and how we can create the repeatedly mentioned optimal symbiosis based on this experience.

This was a very rapid survery of the problems concerned. Most of them are treated in more detail in my book published by World Scientific in 1991, entitled Computer Epistemology, and many further references can be found in that. Several experiences were collected in a decade-long research in robot vision. The goal was restricted to the identification of a pre-determined but easily teachable class of well-defined artificial objects as tools, machine parts.

The other projects mentioned are expert systems which use a combination of logic and pattern recognition. The first one is well-advanced in practice and is directed to the early diagnosis and therapy of defects in the newborns' central neural system. This is a computer support for the method developed by Prof. Katona. The other is a support system in legal-administrative decision-making, a task which combines logical procedures and even more subjective, human points of views.

Correspondence: T. Vámos, Computer and Automation Institute, Hungarian Academy of Science, Kende u. 13-17, H-1111 Budapest, Hungary.

B. L. Bauer, D. Hellwig (eds.)

Minimally Invasive Neurosurgery I

(Acta Neurochirurgica / Supplementum 54)

1992. With 113 partly coloured figures. VII, 98 pages.
Cloth DM 150,-, öS 1050,-
Reduced price for subscribers to "Acta Neurochirurgica":
Cloth DM 135,-, öS 945,-
ISBN 3-211-82321-2

Prices are subject to change without notice

Minimally invasive surgical interventions by means of endoscopes have gained in importance and have been recently introduced in neurosurgery. The book gives an extended overview about the applications of endoscopy in modern neurosurgical practice.

The anatomy and topographical relationships of the intracranial cavities and the pathological changes in these areas, especially of the ventricular system, are described.

Different types of flexible and rigid endoscopes and the instrumentation to handle these tools for neurosurgical purposes are introduced. The indications for endoscopic neurosurgical operative procedures include endoscopic stereotactic interventions, evaluations of intracerebral hematomas, cysts, and brain abscesses as well as endoscopic brain tumor surgery. This book gives the first comprehensive synopsis of this new and exciting field.

Contents: J. Lang: Topographic Anatomy of Preformed Intracranial Spaces. - V.B. Karakhan: Endofiberscopic Intracranial Stereotopography and Endofiberscopic Neurosurgery. - H.-D. Reidenbach: Technological Fundamentals of Endoscopic Haemostasis. - L.M. Auer: Ultrasound Stereotaxic Endoscopy in Neurosurgery. - S.K. Powers: Fenestration of Intraventricular Cysts Using a Flexible, Steerable Endoscope. - K. Yamakawa, T. Kondo, M. Yoshioka, and K. Takakura: Application of Superfine Fiberscope for Endovasculoscopy, Ventriculoscopy, and Myeloscopy. - H.M. Mayer, M. Brock, H.-P. Berlien, and B. Weber, Percutaneous Endoscopic Laser Discectomy (PELD). A New Surgical Technique for Non-sequestrated Lumbar Discs. - N. Huewel, A. Perneczky, V. Urban, and G. Fries: Neuroendoscopic Technique for the Operative Treatment of Septated Syringomyelia. - D. Hellwig and B.L. Bauer: Minimally Invasive Neurosurgery by Means of Ultrathin Endoscopes. - L. Zamorano, C. Chavantes, M. Dujovny, G. Malik, and J. Ausman: Stereotactic Endoscopic Interventions in Cystic and Intraventricular Brain Lesions. - F. Hor, M. Desgeorges, and G.L. Rosseau: Tumour Resection by Stereotactic Laser Endoscopy. - A. Camacho and P.J. Kelly: Volumetric Stereotactic Resection of Superficial and Deep Seated Intraaxial Brain Lesions. - E.R. Heikkinen: "Whole Body" Stereotaxy: Application of Stereotactic Endoscopy to Operations of Herniated Lumbar Discs. - A.L. Benabid, S. Lavallee, D. Hoffmann, P. Cinquin, J. Demongeot, and F. Danel: Potential Use of Robots in Endoscopic Neurosurgery. - Subject Index.

*In preparation: **Minimally Invasive Neurosurgery II***

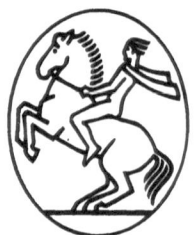

Springer-Verlag Wien New York